Chasing the Gender Dream

Chasing the Gender Dream

The Complete Guide to Conceiving Pink or Blue
With the Latest Sex Selection Technology and Tips
From Someone Who Has Been There

Jennifer Merrill Thompson

ᗡP
Aventine Press

Published by Aventine Press
1202 Donax Ave Suite 12
Imperial Beach, CA 91932, USA
www.aventinepress.com

Library of Congress Cataloging-in-Publication Data
2004103403

ISBN: 1-59330-148-0
Printed in the United States of America

Acknowledgments

I wish to thank my family for putting up with my gender selection obsession, for letting me go on about my daughter preoccupations and for living through my craziness. My loving gratitude to Eddie for agreeing to all the attempts we did, for assisting me in many ways, for contributing his very valuable part and for helping me bring Rachel into this world. There is no greater gift.

Thanks to Jacob and Lucas for being my wonderful little boys, whom I will always love just as much as any girl, including Rachel. You are both very special. Thank you, Jacob, for first making me a mother and for letting me see how much I can instantly love someone I just met, and for being the sweetest little guy. Thank you, Lucas, for being funny and adorable and affectionate, and the absolute best middle child someone can have.

Thank you, Rachel, for coming into this world and letting me be a girl mommy. We will have so much fun together. We already are, with the hair clips and bows. Thank you for wearing pink.

Thanks to all my "board buddies"—you know who you are. If it weren't for you, I never would have felt like there was anybody else who had the same passionate goal as me. We have shared so much. And thanks to those who helped me to learn about IVF and who gave me tips on making those shots less of an "ouch!" My online friends are priceless, and I am so glad I "met" all of you.

Thanks to everyone who shared their story with me for this book, and to those who provided important information. I couldn't have done the book without you.

Thank you to Candice for being one of my few real-life friends who knew what I was going through, and to offer to proofread my book. You're great!

Thank you to MicroSort, and the doctors and nurses at Genetics & IVF Institute, who helped me to reach my dream. Thank you to Dr. Edward Fugger for first envisioning this possibility, and for making it all happen.

Thanks to everyone who was involved in my gender selection journey. It was a long one, but one I would go through again in a heartbeat.

Contents

Preface

For me, this book is about just what it's titled: chasing a gender dream. It grew out of an obsession—an obsession that lasted over the years. I wanted a daughter. My obsession, my chasing the gender dream, took me down every avenue of research, through every book on the subject (and there aren't many) and into every related website. I talked, or e-mailed, with dozens of women on this subject, joined message boards and chat rooms, and made friends (some virtual, some in real life) with people who had a similar obsession.

Most of us did not let people in the real world know of our obsession, our endless quest for a daughter (or, in some cases, a son)—and it was a relief to find other people who felt the same way we did. I met other women who understood my desire to have a daughter to relate to; I was never into sports and "boy" things, and I wanted a chance to raise another female. When family members and friends didn't understand our feelings, it was heartening to meet others who were just like us in this regard: who cherished their children, loved their sons, wouldn't trade them for anyone in the world, but still could not give up the dream for a daughter. It was almost as if something was missing, that there was a little void in our lives that would be filled once our family was complete, once it was balanced with both pink and blue.

This book is about completing that family, about filling that void. And although those of us who try gender selection understand that health is extremely important—and who doesn't want a healthy baby?—we also don't have to apologize for wanting something more, for hoping to influence gender. For those people who tell us, "You are lucky you have healthy children. Don't you think that's enough?" I say, yes, that is very important, but we can't help our longing, can't help wanting to try something to help us find our dream. *Chasing the Gender Dream* is the result of years of research and about personal experience, both mine and others. I write about my own hits and misses, my various attempts at gender selection, and my ultimate success at bringing a girl into our family after two boys, after almost giving up on the idea. It's also about other people's stories; I write about women who have tried both low-tech (home methods) and high-tech (laboratory methods) to fulfill their gender dreams. I discuss what people are doing in the way of gender preconception diets. I have taken every tip and method I've heard about, whether it's proven or not, and included it in this book. Most of the methods do not provide a 100 percent guarantee of success, but I include them all here, so that everything out there on gender selection can be found in one place. I also include medical and professional opinions wherever I can, and I try to provide the latest information on fertility technologies.

If I've missed a method or left out a particular type of clinic, it's not intentional. I am writing about the most well-known techniques I've heard and read about. Instead of searching all over the globe for some answers, as I did, you can find a thorough summary here of what many people have tried. And if you've heard about some of these methods, and are curious about what they're like (especially with using the new MicroSort technology), I hope that my experiences, and others, will help you make the decision on whether or not to go that particular route. Let me be your guinea pig!

One note: A majority of this book is about trying to conceive a girl, rather than a boy. This comes from two reasons: (1) my own personal experience at female sex selection, and (2) my discovery that people who are looking to influence gender are most often trying for a girl. As a result, there seem to be more girl methods. But I also try to include everything I've learned about gender selection for boys in this book.

Finally, I understand that sex selection is controversial, and it may continue to be for a long time. I hope that more and more people will understand the value of these methods, and not disparage us, realizing how much our lives can be enriched by successful gender selection, by "family balancing." It is wonderful to be able to experience raising both a son and a daughter.

My journey truly changed my life—it brought me my daughter, Rachel. And I hope I can help you.

CHAPTER

1

Dreaming in Pink or Blue

"I've always wanted a daughter."

This is a dream of many women—an image of a baby in pink, of a little girl to dress up and to mold into a young woman, of a female to relate to, someone who will share that mother-daughter bond and may follow in her mom's footsteps.

"We've been hoping to have a son, to carry on the family name."

Maybe the longing is for a little boy. Some men harbor an image of a son in the family, a hope for a boy to play sports with and to teach, a young man to have pride in and to raise to adulthood.

"With each pregnancy, we hope to have the opposite gender. But I guess it will never happen."

Some couples continue to have child after child of the same gender, taking their chances that the pattern will change and that maybe they will conceive a baby of the opposite sex. Some will, but many will not.

"We only want two children, and we'd like to experience both a son and a daughter."

Maybe a couple wants the chance to achieve the hope of a "balanced" family, of both blue and pink. This is a common scenario. It is priceless to have the opportunity to raise both a little boy *and* a little girl. And with smaller families planned nowadays, there isn't as much time to wait for both to come to a couple.

How far are these people willing to go to achieve their dream? What would they do to reach that sought-after picture of a little girl or a little boy in their home? How much of their hard-earned money would they be willing to invest? Would they want to "play" with nature?

Would you?

I did. And the result was a beautiful little girl after two wonderful boys: a pregnancy that might never have happened for me if I had let nature take its course—a pregnancy in which I finally saw the "three white lines" on the sonogram screen at 20 weeks gestation, an image that I had longed for and almost given up on as possible for my family.

What if you could do something *before* your baby was conceived to increase your chances of a certain gender? What if this option was not just a shot in the dark, pursuing a theory you've heard of or trying an old wives' tale at home—but, actually, a high-tech method of helping two people conceive a little boy or a little girl? Would you do it? It now is possible. And more couples nowadays are considering it.

The Natural Odds

Many people have heard that if a couple has two children, both of the same gender, their chances of conceiving a third child of the same gender are higher than that of the opposite gender. Basically, if a family has two boys, no girls, and they're expecting another child, they can count on another boy instead of a girl, according to the statistics. A family with three girls can probably expect another girl in the next pregnancy. No one knows for sure why that is, except that there might be something inherent in the father or mother, or both, that favors the conception of one gender over another.

Some studies have shown that the odds of conceiving the opposite gender go down with each subsequent birth of the original gender. (In other words, the more girls a couple have, the less likely they are to conceive a boy.) In one study of 150,000 births in the United States, researchers Yoram Ben-Porath and Finis Welch found that the sex ratio (percentage of male babies over female babies) of a current birth given no previous brothers and zero, one, two, three or four previous sisters was 51.3, 50.1, 49.2, 48.6 and 45.1 percent, respectively (published in the *Quarterly Journal of Economics*, May 1976, Vol. 90). So the couple's chances go down with each birth.

As a result of these statistics, it may be hard for couples to "beat the odds" if they really want a child of the opposite gender. Yes, they could try pregnancy after pregnancy, and maybe they'll be lucky. But if not, this ends up being a large, costly undertaking—a big family is very expensive to care for, to raise and to finance for college.

Some other studies have shown that couples with "mixed" genders—both boys and girls—are less likely to continue to grow their families. They are more apt to stop with fewer children. Couples with all-gender offspring, on the other hand, are more likely to continue to have more kids, hoping that the next one might be the opposite gender. I personally have known families that fit that description.

One study that shows this phenomenon was published in the journal *Human Reproduction*. Researchers at Denmark's Centre for Research in Health & Social Statistics analyzed the effect of sex combination of previously born children in the family on fertility rates for more than 360,000 Danish families (with a total of 613,900 children), to address the questions of sex preference and combination preference. They state that the fertility rates were stratified by parental age and the latency time to the next child, and fertility rate ratios were estimated.

"Our results demonstrate a strong preference for a balanced composition of sexes in Danish families," the researchers reported in *Human Reproduction*'s April 1999 issue (Vol. 14). "In families with two or three children, the highest fertility rates were seen in families who had same-sexed children. The lowest fertility rates were in families with two children of identical sex followed by a child of the opposite sex. A moderate sex preference for girls was indicated by higher fertility rates in two-boy families than in two-girl families."

This study confirms that many couples are interested in balancing the genders in their family. Most would like both a boy and a girl. Sometimes nature easily provides this, and sometimes it doesn't.

New Trends in Families

A significant factor that plays into the increased demand for gender selection these days may be the trend of more women putting off starting a family. Some working women, who perhaps concentrated on their careers throughout their 20s and much of their 30s, have waited to have children. For those who wait until their mid or late 30s, they may be lucky to have one or two children as it is, as fertility definitely declines after age 35.

Over the past three decades, the average age for American women to have their first baby has increased by almost four years (from 21.4 years in 1970 to almost 25 years in 2000), and the average age of mothers for all births rose almost three years (from 24.6 years to 27.2 years), according to the Center for Disease Control's National Center for Health Statistics (NCHS). It will probably continue to rise. Over one-half of all births still occur to women in their 20s—the peak childbearing years—but the average age in this group has shifted steadily upward since 1970, according to NCHS.

"The increase in the average age of women having a baby also reflects the relatively recent downturn in the teen birth rate and the rising birth rates for women in their 30s and 40s," according to NCHS, which bases its report on birth certificates filed in state vital statistics offices. "The trend in delayed childbirth is universal—observed nationwide and among all groups in the population." With women waiting longer to start having children, the family size inevitably will be smaller. And what if a couple really wants one of those children to be a girl? Or a boy? Enter gender selection technology, which will substantially increase a couple's chances of a desired gender. Now, instead of having boy after boy, or girl after girl, in the quest for the "other" sex—or if a couple is only able to have one or two children because of maternal age—parents can invest the money into a medical procedure that brings them closer to their goal. And it doesn't involve a folk remedy or a "magical" potion, but something much more connected to science. That is what we did, and after a long journey, it worked.

The Technology

My husband and I used the new technology of MicroSort, which is sperm sorting using *flow cytometric separation* of X (female) and Y (male) chromosome-bearing sperm cells. After the separation, the resulting sort is used to impregnate the woman. This originally had been done with livestock; now it's in FDA clinical trials for humans. It is the only method that seems to be given any validation in the medical journals, the only technique that seems to have true scientific backing, especially for the preselection of female babies.

"Nothing worked until now," Dr. Alan DeCherney, chairperson of obstetrics and gynecology at the University of California at Los Angeles and the editor of the journal *Fertility and Sterility*, told the *New York Times* when the news about MicroSort was first coming out. Since 1995, MicroSort has been drawing couples from all over the country (and some from across the world) to its Fairfax, Va., headquarters to participate in the clinical study.

MicroSort gives women a greater than 90 percent chance of a baby girl if they're fortunate enough to get pregnant. And it is the method that finally worked for us—and possibly could work for you. The MicroSort clinic is a division of the Genetics & IVF Institute. Until 2002, the Fairfax clinic was the only place in the world to offer this technology, but MicroSort West then opened at the Huntington Reproductive Center of Southern California, offering West Coast families a chance at this technology closer to home. Someday, when MicroSort is out of clinical trials and open for widespread licensing, it should be offered at clinics all over the country, and possibly the world.

For patients who are accepted into the MicroSort program, their sorted sperm specimens are used to achieve a pregnancy with either intrauterine insemination or in-vitro fertilization. We tried both, and those details will come later in this book. But first, we'll take a look at many of the other methods that are attempted for gender selection.

And maybe *you* could be one step closer to that little girl (or boy) that you've always dreamed of having.

CHAPTER

2

The Methods Up Until Now

Throughout time, people have tried everything they could think of to influence the sex of their future children. Gender has meant a lot to parents—the single biggest characteristic, after health, of a new baby. In places such as China and India, a boy baby historically has brought joy; a girl baby, the opposite, and sometimes selective abortion or infanticide has, tragically, resulted. In many countries, women who bring sons into the world are honored and feted; it is considered a great accomplishment for the family. In the United States, on the other hand, there appears to be more interest in trying to conceive a girl—maybe because of American women's increased roles and rights, their ability to say what they want and to "go for it," and they often want daughters.

The history of attempting gender preselection has some very classical beginnings.

"The Hebrew Talmud suggested that placing the marriage bed in a north-south direction favored the conception of boys," according to Gale Largey in *Encyclopedia of Bioethics* (1978). In Germany, if a couple wanted a boy, the man was advised to take an ax to bed with him at night. Other suggestions for influencing a baby's gender "included having intercourse in dry weather or when there is a north wind; having the man wear boots to bed or hanging his pants on the right bedpost; or having the woman lie on her right side during intercourse or wear male clothing to bed on her wedding night," according to Loras College's Catholic Healthcare Ethics.

"To get a boy, the men of ancient Greece had sex while lying on their right side. Their counterparts in 18th-century France actually tied off their left testicle to attain a male child," wrote Virginia Gilbert in an online article at Preconception.com. "And according to classical Chinese theory, a woman could choose her baby's gender even into the third month of pregnancy: handling pearls would bring a girl; holding a bow and arrow, a boy," wrote Gilbert.

Well, we all know now that gender is determined at conception, not afterward. But what we can do *before* that conception is the issue that some people are preoccupied with now.

With every year that goes by, new gender myths and "methods" are conceived and attempted. From timing conception during a certain part of a women's ovulatary cycle, to trying gender "diets" and supplements, to special douching, it is amazing the lengths that people will go to try to control the timeless act of conception—to try to produce a baby girl or a baby boy. But it is understandable. I've tried most of them.

The Shettles Method

Many have read Dr. Landrum B. Shettles' *How to Choose the Sex of Your Baby* (first published in 1989) and tried his method of timing intercourse (and other things) to increase the chance of a certain gender. This is one of the many "at-home" methods—and the most well-known—that people can try. It has worked for some couples; others have gotten an "opposite" result. Shettles' book has been revised a few times (most recently in 1997) and some of his steps have been updated, but the basic point the book makes is that calculating the time of the woman's ovulation—and then attempting conception during certain times of her cycle—is the most important aspect of trying for a certain gender.

The idea is that male-chromosome-carrying sperm move faster but don't last as long as the bigger, hardier female-chromosome-carrying sperm. For a boy baby, the couple should aim at timing sex on the day of ovulation, or the day before; for a girl, the couple should try a few days before ovulation. (This timing for a girl baby is quite difficult, and women are recommended to track their cycles for several months in advance to pinpoint their normal time of ovulation.)

The late Dr. Shettles was an obstetrician-gynecologist who was an acknowledged pioneer in the field of in-vitro fertilization. In his book he encourages women to use the cervical mucus method for detecting ovulation (daily examining discharge from the cervix and noticing the differences during different times of the cycle). There also is the taking of basal body temperature (BBT), a process done first thing in the morning before getting out of bed; this helps determine your current place in the monthly cycle. Usually a woman will notice a temperature dip before ovulation, and then a sharp rise afterward. I always kept a monthly BBT chart on graph paper and it helped me see my menstrual patterns. And, if you're willing to put out some cash, you can buy ovulation predictor kits at the drugstore; these also help with cycle monitoring. I bought my share of those when trying these at-home methods. (And for a great book on fertility awareness, check out Toni Weschler's *Taking Charge of Your Fertility*; this book really helps women figure out what their body is doing during different times of the menstrual/ovulatory cycle.)

Shettles also discusses the use of alkaline (for a boy) and acidic (for a girl) douches to enhance gender methods and he advises on the correct ways to use them. Some women insert these vaginal douches before intercourse, in hopes of providing the correct internal environment for the particular sperm they want to attract. An alkaline reproductive tract is supposedly more amenable to the faster, smaller male sperm, whereas an acidic tract kills off the weaker males and gives the slower but hardier female sperm a better chance at surviving and penetrating the host egg when it arrives.

These are all good ideas if they work, and some women have had great success stories with trying one or a combination of these techniques. For me, unfortunately, I never could get pregnant using the Shettles method. After months of tracking my cycle and then months of aiming a few days before ovulation to get pregnant, we ended up getting closer and closer to ovulation in our futile attempts, and eventually got pregnant with our second son, right around what I believe was my ovulation day. Lucas (like his older brother) is one of the lights of my life, and in no way did I ever regret conceiving him or want to trade him for any baby girl in the world. But for us, using Shettles to conceive a daughter was just too difficult.

A Shettles Success Story

Such difficulty wasn't the case, however, for Susan in California. After three boys, two of them twins, she used Shettles timing and lots of other ideas to get her girl. She read Dr. Shettles' book, joined some Internet message boards (at the Baby Center and iVillage's Parent Soup—see appendix) and researched everything she could find.

When Susan was 31, she conceived her daughter. She had been monitoring her monthly cycles and gotten to know them very well, by using daily ovulation predictor strips (which she bought cheaply online), taking her temperature every morning, and charting her cervical mucus as well as her cervical position (the cervix supposedly moves higher or lower according to which part of the ovulatory cycle a woman is in).

In addition, "I had switched to a vegetarian diet (no meat at all) three months prior to trying to conceive. I read in a women's magazine that in a study in Britain, there were something like

102 girls to 100 boys in vegetarian moms. That was good enough for me!" Susan laughs. "I also had cut back on salt and was taking calcium supplements and eating lots of extra calcium."

In that "fateful month," Susan took cranberry tablets (which are believed to acidify the reproductive tract) three times a day for two weeks leading up to ovulation. "The few days before ovulating, I also took Sudafed, which helped not just my allergy symptoms, but dried up my cervical mucus."

Susan and her husband also decided to abstain from sex in the days prior to their baby attempt. She says that with their previous children, they had had intercourse every day when trying to conceive. This time, "I hoped that the abstinence might kill off some of the weaker 'Y' sperm."

Their plan was to have just one act of intercourse three days before Susan ovulated, as per the Shettles method for a girl. It ended up being a 2½ -day cutoff.

"We did many sentimental and superstitious things as well," Susan confides. "I filled our bedroom with pink flowers, lit pink candles, put a pink baby outfit under the bed, even wore pink underwear and bra, and I painted my toenails pink.

"I prayed my heart out! I wanted the conception of her to be a memorable one, and it is neat to know exactly how and when it happened. We did a missionary position, very, very shallow penetration [both touted as more conducive to conceiving girls), and I lay there for a couple of minutes. That was it!"

Susan's twin boys were 5½ and her youngest son was almost 1 when she conceived her daughter. "Truly, I mostly credit God answering my prayers, but I also analyzed and researched what I did with my other pregnancies and tried almost the opposite this last time. I also used anecdotes from other women on the Gender Determination board at Parent Soup and followed my heart!"

Asked how long it took her to get pregnant with her daughter, she says, blushing, "The first month we tried."

"Since having a daughter, I have felt many waves of appreciation that I am raising both genders. She is 17 months old now, and we play with tea sets, cuddle her dolls and shop for feminine clothes. I also cherish the way I can picture her growing into a young woman one day, and one day talking with her about topics that are unique to women, from carrying a baby, to being strong and confident as a woman, and being proud of her beauty without having that be what her self-image is based upon."

The Whelan Method: Opposing Shettles

Susan's efforts all paid off. Or was it just going to happen anyway? There is no way to know for sure. There are a lot of differing opinions on the validity of at-home sex selection. Another book, Elizabeth Whelan's *Boy or Girl?*, disputes the Shettles method and actually suggests the opposite in timing conception. Whelan recommends that because of biochemical changes that may favor male-producing sperm early in a woman's cycle, couples desiring a boy should have intercourse four to six days before their BBT goes up. If they want a girl, abstaining from sex until a couple days before ovulation is the recommended course.

Whelan is reported to have predicted that this method has a 68 percent success rate for boy baby-making, and just 56 percent for girl baby-making. It is still better than the 50/50 odds most couples naturally have, but I personally have never heard of anyone who has tried this method. Most women whom I have surveyed, of those trying home methods of gender selection, have gone the Shettles route (about half to success, half not).

A Case of Persistence

Ellie in Sydney, Australia, would not give up on the timing methods proposed by Dr. Shettles. She tried his suggested timing for four of her five children before she finally got the daughter she had wanted for so long. She had sons who were 8, 6, 3 and 1 when she conceived a girl at age 34.

"I set out to try Shettles with the last three of the boys but always ended up becoming impatient and just throwing caution to the wind in the end," she says. "I suppose I thought if I had four kids altogether, one was bound to be a girl. Of course I was wrong!"

Before conceiving her daughter, Ellie did three practice cycles and then actively tried to become pregnant, succeeding on her third month of trying. She also stuck to a very strict gender diet that was low in sodium and potassium and high in calcium and magnesium.

Life with a daughter has been everything she had hoped. "I feel such an inner peace to finally have a daughter to go along with my wonderful sons," Ellie says. "I love the way my boys now get to relate to another female in the family instead of everything being so male-dominated all the time. I feel happy and thankful every day for a dream come true." Her little girl turned 2 in August 2003.

Additional At-Home Techniques

Besides using Shettles timing and a gender diet as Ellie and Susan did (and more about diets in the next chapter), many women try other sex selection tips. Following are some of those ideas (though in no way are any of them a guarantee of success!).

- **Sex position:** for a baby girl, have sexual intercourse in the missionary position; for a baby boy, try other positions, such as the woman on top.

- **Acidity vs. alkalinity:** for a baby girl, some women eat or douche with lemon (or vinegar) to increase their environmental acidity; women trying for a boy avoid lemon and other acidic foods and may douche with baking soda. Many women have a vaginal environment that is naturally either more acidic or more alkaline. Some have actually tested their body's pH levels (there are products available on the Internet for this).
- **Penetration at intercourse:** for a baby girl, a couple should have shallow penetration during sex; for a boy, deep penetration is advised. This theory is due to the fact that the secretions of the cervix are believed to be less acidic than those of the vagina. Also, anything that makes it more difficult for the sperm to travel up the reproductive tract is supposed to make a conception more conducive for producing a girl.
- **Orgasm:** for a baby girl, no orgasm for the woman during an attempted conception; for a baby boy, female orgasm may help push the smaller boy sperm along. It also is said to help alter the acidity/alkalinity level of the female reproductive tract.
- **Testes temperature:** for a baby girl, heating up the male's genitals is supposed to help (the warmer it is, the more likely he supposedly can conceive a girl, though this also decreases fertility); for the reverse, a cooler area will help, and looser underwear (boxers instead of briefs). Men wanting sons should avoid taking a hot bath or soaking in a hot tub; for daughters, some couples try this before intercourse.
- **Cervical fluids:** for a baby girl, decreased fluids make it harder for the less hardy male-producing sperm to swim through the woman's reproductive tract, favoring the stronger female sperm; increased fluids help for boy babies. As a result, some women who want boys have reportedly

taken the cold medicine Benadryl to increase their cervical fluid and help usher the boy sperm along. Women who want girls try to dry up their cervical mucus (taking the oral fertility medicine Clomid has been known to do this, thus agreeing with the theory that more women on Clomid produce girls). There are a variety of ways to try to dry up the mucus. Also, different parts of a woman's monthly cycle cause different stages in mucus production, and some women are naturally wetter or drier than others!

- **Supplements:** for a baby girl, cranberry tablets have been used as a special gender supplement; the reverse would be true for baby boys.
- **Got milk?** Women who are big milk drinkers may have more girls; those who avoid milk may see more boys. At least that's one of the theories!

The Moon, the Chinese Birth Chart and More

In addition to the preceding sex selection tips, some people believe that the gender of a child is determined by the position of the moon at conception. Although there is no scientific evidence that this lunar method is true, every year this theory gets brought up and some couples attempt it. Czech psychiatrist and gynecologist Eugene Jonas examined the idea of the natal lunar fertile phase in the 1950s, and his ideas still are used today for both fertility and for gender determination. Dr. Jonas reportedly discovered a fertility cycle that is determined by the angular relationship between the sun and moon at the time of a woman's birth.

Each month, when this angle is repeated, fertility is supposed to be at its peak. And, the story goes, the gender of a future baby can be determined based on the sign the moon occupied at the moment of conception. If the moon was in a positive sign when the sun/moon angle recurred, the child would be a boy; if the moon was in a negative sign, the child would be a girl.

And then there's the ancient Chinese birth chart. Although I never gave this theory any consideration (or, for that matter, the lunar method), some people do put stock into it and say it has worked for them. It also is related to moon changes. Legend has it that a Chinese birth chart (supposedly predicting the gender of a baby with 93 percent accuracy) was buried in a tomb near Beijing for almost 700 years (and is now located at the Beijing Institute of Science). For women who are already pregnant, they can find out if the chart predicts that their baby will be a boy or a girl. And if they're trying to conceive and would like to maximize their chances of a particular gender, they are recommended to use the chart as a guide to the best month for getting pregnant. The chart predicts the gender of an unborn child based on the mother's age and the month of conception.

"One theory explaining the chart is that a woman's secretions change lunar month by lunar month, either more acidic or alkaline according to her lunar age," according to an organization called ChinaGold. "This change decides which sperm are favored for that lunar month." ChinaGold did a survey using more than 4,100 conception dates and came up with an accuracy rate of 65 percent for the Chinese chart. (For more information, the organization's website is listed in this book's appendix.)

Undoubtedly, there are a lot of ideas floating around that people have tried. (For another possible idea, see the adjacent box, "Parental Age and Gender.") Women have attempted all of the above at-home tips, and more. The list seems to get longer every day. Go to an Internet forum, and you may learn more details about the above tips, or even more ideas. (For example, check out the online "Gender Determination" message board at iVillage's Parent Soup.)

Parental Age and Gender

An additional factor cited for conceiving baby girls is advanced maternal or paternal age—although there is not much you can do about this to increase your odds except wait until you and your spouse are older! Some research has shown that younger men with higher sperm counts may make more boys, while the older that parents are (and thus the less fertile) at conception, the higher the chances they will produce girls. Women in their 40s may be more likely to conceive a girl than a boy (although it's not always the case).

In one study, a team of epidemiologists from New Jersey, using more than 20 years of birth reports, concluded that parental age is related to the percentage of total births of each gender. As reported in the journal *Fertility and Sterility* (March 2000, Vol. 73), having older parents is specifically associated with a higher percentage of female newborns. The researchers (Nicholich et al.) noted a downward trend in the male birth fraction over the years—finding that parental age is one of the most prominent variables in this.

In my own extended family, I have seen what looks like evidence of this theory: In five pregnancies in which the mother was 40 or older, all five babies (from five separate women) ended up being girls—even in two cases in which there were three boys, or four, preceding the only girl!

So the longer you wait, the more of a chance there may be that you conceive a daughter.

The Chance of Failure

All of the above low-tech methods of gender selection have their proponents, and they certainly are not costly, invasive or jeopardizing of privacy (as the high-tech methods can be).

But, of course, there is no guarantee with any of them. And, very important: the couple attempting gender selection have to be prepared to embrace either gender, whatever that baby they're conceiving turns out to be. There could very likely be a gender selection "failure" (although the baby, of course, is not a failure).

If the child conceived turns out to be the opposite of the gender tried for, those parents must be ready to welcome and love that little being above everything. I think that is generally understood. But the reality, when it hits, can bring out a lot of emotion. I know I cried for a while after my second baby's ultrasound when I found out I was carrying another boy. I so wanted a daughter, and I was envious of other women having baby girls. But after a while I adjusted to the idea and got excited to meet my little son and to give my 2-year-old, Jacob, a younger brother. But it's not always an easy adjustment, especially when you've put a lot of time and effort into trying for a certain gender only to be disappointed (at least initially). Some parents go through an emotional wringer.

Meg, 32, lived in Denver with her husband and two young sons and read up on everything she could find to learn how to produce the daughter she had longed for with a passion. She read Dr. Shettles' book and tried all of his recommendations, including douching and "all the bells and whistles." When she got pregnant, she was sure she was successful and waited anxiously for the ultrasound to confirm her hope of a girl. But first she got major news: she was carrying twins. Some weeks later, she found out they were both boys. She was devastated.

Meg became angry that the methods did not work for her, depressed that she was going to be the mother of four boys, and desperate about the fact that she would never have a girl. Four children were the limit for her and her husband. She soon went into a spiral of despair that tainted her pregnancy and fogged her days. She couldn't give her two sons the attention they needed. She even considered putting up the twins for adoption once they were born. It was only after she got into therapy that her life started to brighten and she learned to accept the idea of being mother to four boys. It was a long road for her to get back to some semblance of happiness. And, of course, the rest of her family suffered as well. For Meg, maybe gender selection was not something to pursue.

Roll of the Dice?

The success rate for the Shettles timing method is unpredictable. Different surveys come up with different results. Dr. Shettles, before his death in February 2003, would tell you that his method increases your chances of a desired gender (especially if you're trying for a boy, which has better success rates). Others claim the technique does not work—that just as many "opposites" result as babies of the tried-for gender. In 1984, the World Health Organization published a study that it says failed to confirm a gender predominance in relation to the timing of conception.

So the Shettles method is not considered a surefire way to conceive gender. But every year, couples continue to try his methods. Some conceive the gender they're seeking; some do not. Maybe it depends on how successfully they follow all his instructions and tips. And some couples try some of the numerous other techniques along with the Shettles timing. But people may try everything and still end up with the same gender they had before, as if they had tried nothing at all.

But if you're willing to accept and love unequivocally a gender "opposite," then trying the gender selection methods may be for you. As Meg found out, no at-home method is a definite means to a girl baby or boy baby. If you're up for the challenge, have the drive and determination to see it through and can handle the possible disappointment of conceiving an "opposite," it may be worth it to attempt some of these methods. And read on for more!

CHAPTER

3

The Diet Alternative

What if what you ate made a difference in the type of children you produced? More specifically, what if your preconception diet affected their gender?

In recent years, theories have come up about parents' everyday diets being a possible precursor to the gender of their children. Certain ideas have emerged—such as vegetarian or high-calcium diets for producing girls, and diets with plenty of meat and sodium for boys—and some of these theories are being taken seriously.

While in some cases conclusions were drawn from looking at the genders of children of people who, for example, normally drank lots of milk, other people specifically focused on *changing* their preconception diets to influence gender, usually the opposite gender of what their current children were. In most cases, it is the prospective mother who follows a particular "gender diet."

Thirty years ago, a study suggested that a woman's internal environment may have something to do with fetal gender. According to R. Revelle in the *New England Journal of Medicine,* "data suggest that spermatozoa carrying X and Y chromosomes respond differently to at least some differences in environmental conditions" (1974, Vol. 291, No. 20). The data came from a study on the type and time of insemination within the menstrual cycle with the human sex ratio at birth.

If the woman's environment, or pH levels, can possibly influence the response of her partner's X and Y sperm during or after intercourse, then does it follow that what the woman eats may affect her inclination for boy or girl conceptions?

Well, there is mixed opinion on this, as there are on most gender preselection methods. Some researchers believe there is some credibility to the theories; others do not. Either way, many gender diets have cropped up for those who want to give this idea a whirl. Most of the diets I have seen are basically similar, and often the general idea is that eating certain foods makes a woman's reproductive tract more hospitable to girl sperm if it's made more acidic and to boy sperm if alkalinity is increased. Diet proponents usually recommend having the person start the diet at least six weeks before trying to conceive a child in the desired gender. Some experts recommend certain supplements as well, such as calcium or cranberry tablets for a girl (as mentioned in the previous chapter). I tried a bit of a "girl" diet, and I have to tell you it was difficult! Taking supplements is the easy part.

The Vegetarian Theory

Are you thinking of going meatless? Can giving up meat help you to conceive a baby girl? This is a relatively new theory, and a recent British study may back up the idea. In what may be the first study of its kind, researchers at Nottingham University in England followed more than 5,000 pregnant women and found significant differences in the gender of babies born to vegetarian and non-vegetarian mothers. The study involved data from British midwives, and the findings were published in the British journal *Practising Midwife* (2000, Vol. 3, No. 7).

Among the study's statistically significant results, it was found that the gender ratio of male-to-female babies for vegetarians was 81.5 to 100; this is compared against a British national ratio of 106 to 100.

"This was an incidental finding," according to a statement that researcher Pauline Hudson told BBC News Online. "We had been looking at the impact of diet on baby weight. But it is not something we have published lightly; this was a very well-carried-out study."

The researchers extended their initial study for another six months and looked at only the sex of babies. The results were similar.

Hudson told the BBC that the mechanism behind the impact of diet was unclear, but she put forward three possible theories: (1) a vegetarian diet places stress on the female body, meaning that female fetuses, which are known to be more robust, survive, while male fetuses die off; (2) a vegetarian diet changes the acidity of the vaginal secretions, creating a hostile environment for sperm carrying male genetic information; and (3) the diet contains chemicals that mimic the action of female sex hormones such as estrogen.

Hudson and Rosemary Buckley, who reported the study results in *The Practising Midwife,* comment, "The lack of meat and fish in the vegetarian diet and the high intakes of dairy produce, eggs and nuts that are a feature of vegetarian diets may account for the difference in the sex ratio."

Vegetarian Economy & Green Agriculture, a British charitable organization that followed the study, adds, "Other studies of preconception diets and their effects on the gender ratio indicate the following influences from the mother's diet: to conceive boys, high intakes of salt, meat, fish, jams, dried vegetables, wine and beer are recommended, with avoidance of milk, whole-meal bread, spinach and mustard; to conceive a girl, the diet should be high in dairy produce, eggs, nuts and clementine oranges, with avoidance of tea, coffee, wine, fish fingers, cheese, oranges and peaches."

Mineral Intakes

More diet advice comes from Sue Roebuck, a fertility management and reproductive health advisor in Australia, who states that the most important factor of her recommended gender preconception diet is the ratio of potassium to calcium. She encourages participants to consume mineral supplements as well as to follow the diet. "It is believed that the increased intake of these minerals changes the mineral structure of the egg during its ripening stage, and this makes it more receptive to sperm bearing the X-chromosome (girl) or the Y-chromosome (boy)."

Roebuck is on staff at the Energy Health Centre in South Yarra, Melbourne, a clinic that also provides office gender preselection services for local women involving "hormonal assessment during the fertile phase of the cycle" and fertility charts that she has designed.

In addition to providing the gender services, Roebuck recommends patients follow the booklet that she has written, "Choosing Your Baby Through Diet," which details both her boy diet and her girl diet and provides several recipes to help people follow the diet. "Both diets require a lot of determination, motivation and perseverance!" she comments.

Roebuck credits French physiologist Joseph Stolkowski as the founder of the theory of sex selection by diet. A few decades ago, Stolkowski conducted an agricultural experiment involving giving cattle a calcium-enriched feed, according to Roebuck. When the cattle ate a balanced diet, that is, "the proportions of potassium, calcium and magnesium were more or less equal, the ratio of male to female was almost equal—148 males, 149 females."

Roebuck continues, "When calcium enrichment was given with a reduction of sodium, the results showed a marked increase in female births—340 to 280 males. (The adrenal glands, which are affected by sodium, regulate the level of potassium in the body.)"

According to an article in *Parade* magazine (June 27, 1982), Dr. Stolkowski believed that if a couple wanted to conceive a boy, the woman should eat foods rich in potassium and sodium—such as meat, fish, vegetables, chocolate and salt—for at least six weeks before conception time. For a baby girl, she should eat foods rich in calcium and magnesium—such as milk, cheese, nuts, beans and cereals. Dr. Stolkowski's premise was that the determination of baby gender is influenced by ionic factors—that by controlling the ratio of potassium and sodium ions to calcium and magnesium ions, a woman somehow alters her ovarian metabolism. And her internal mineral balance may affect the consistency of her cervical mucus, or some other environmental condition within her reproductive tract, making it more hospitable to one type of sperm or the other, Stolkowski believed.

Roebuck cites a 1975-77 dietary intake study in France following people using the two gender diets, which had trial success rates from 77 to 88 percent, but she comments that the diets were difficult to follow and about two-thirds of participants gave up. She also urges prospective participants to start their diet 6 to 10 weeks before their planned conception, that they have a medical checkup before beginning and that they follow the diets under careful medical supervision. Those with poor kidney function or heart disease should not attempt gender diets.

For more information about Roebuck's "Choosing Your Baby Through Diet," contact the Energy Health Centre, listed in this book's appendix.

Dr. Stolkowski's gender diet tenets have influenced other medical researchers as well. *The Preconception Gender Diet*, a book published in 1982 (see appendix), is based on Stolkowski's reported work. Its authors, Sally Langendoen and William Proctor, also suggest that to conceive a baby girl, a woman should eat a diet low in potassium and sodium, and high in calcium and magnesium; and to conceive a boy, she should increase sodium and potassium, and reduce calcium. They believe that by altering one's diet to include and exclude certain foods, we can directly influence the conditions in the reproductive tract, increasing the odds of conceiving either a boy or a girl. One clinical trial showed an 80 percent accuracy rate for 260 women following the gender diet and using supplements. This study showed no adverse events or reported birth defects.

I have come across this same basic gender diet in several places. One report states that German scientists in 1935 accidentally noticed, while studying the effects of potassium, that an increase in potassium was associated with an increase in male births. According to GeoCities' Gender Determination website, the same results were achieved by other scientists in Germany and France in 1938, 1958, 1967 and 1969 using different types of animals. "They claimed that there was a remarkable increase in females when there is more magnesium and less potassium."

According to those researchers, gender diet can change the pH level in the woman's body and therefore change the polarity of the egg. For conceiving a daughter, the diet depends on increasing magnesium and reducing potassium. To increase magnesium, you need to take in more calcium to help the body with absorption. And if you're trying to conceive a son, you need to increase potassium by taking in more sodium (salt) and to reduce magnesium by avoiding both calcium and magnesium, according to diet proponents.

Preconception Diets

Following are the food guidelines, obtained from GeoCities (listed in appendix), for the preconception girl diet and boy diet:

THE GIRL DIET

Objective: To increase calcium and magnesium while decreasing potassium and sodium in your diet.

Daily recommended supplements:
- Calcium: 800 mg
- Magnesium: 300 mg
- Vitamin D

Daily fluid intake:
- Must be 2–2.5 liters (8–10 glasses)
- Very important for calcium absorption

Milk:
- Drink 750 ml per day (whole, 2 percent, skim, etc.)
- Include two milk products (e.g., yogurt, pudding, custard) each day

Eggs:
- Allowed, but do not introduce forbidden foods (e.g., a cheese omelet)

Cheese:
- Parmesan cheese, one dessert spoon maximum twice a week
- Small servings of cottage cheese

Tea and coffee:
- Basically forbidden, but one cup only of either is acceptable
- It must be very weak

Mineral water:
- Evian, Perrier

Wine:
- An occasional drink allowed (150 ml)

Meat—maximum 130 g per day

Lamb:
- One mid-loin chop (large): 130 g
- One chump chop (average): 130 g
- One forequarter chop: 115–120 g

Beef:
- One piece of oyster blade (medium): 130–150 g
- Half a T-bone steak: 130–150 g
- One piece of eye fillet
- One piece of sandwich steak: 60 g

Pork:
- One butterfly steak: 115–120 g
- One mid-loin (medium): 120 g

Chicken:
- One breast barbecued chicken (family size) and meat from one drumstick: approximately 130 g

Fish:
- Must be cooked in a "court bouillon"—that is, 500 ml water, a little wine or wine vinegar and herbs
  (this reduces the salt content)

Bread:
- Must be low-salt (content less than 1 percent)
- Salt-free crisp-bread (Lanes Premium 50-percent-less salt cracker)

Pasta:
- Permitted without restriction, provided that forbidden ingredients are not involved in the preparation

Rice:
- Brown or white rice allowed

Cereals:
- Semolina, tapioca, corn-flour, flour allowed
- Puffed rice (available at health food stores)

THE BOY DIET

Objective: To increase sodium and potassium while decreasing magnesium and calcium in your diet.

Daily recommended supplements:
- Chlorvescent or Slow K tablets (one tablet to be taken twice daily, morning and evening)
- Potassium supplements (200 mg per day)

Tea and coffee:
- As desired (high in potassium)

Fruit juice:
- 500 ml per day
- Must be 100 percent pure fruit juice
- Do not drink "fruit-based" drinks, as the mineral content is lower
- Fruit cordial occasionally

Mineral water:
- 500 ml per day
- Hepburn Spa and Schweppes are the only permitted brands

Soft drinks:
- Coca Cola, lemonade, tonic water and so forth, as desired (high in sodium and potassium)

Alcohol:
- Wine: 300 ml maximum per day allowed
- Beer and cider: as desired
- Spirits: They have a diuretic effect, which causes excessive excretion of mineral salts

Dairy products: Basically forbidden

Milk:
- Forbidden!
- The soybean beverage Vitasoy is an acceptable alternative to milk when used in cooking—this brand has the lowest calcium content

Butter: Moderate amount only of salted butter

Margarine: Allowed

Cheese: Forbidden

Eggs:
- Whites only allowed
- Best avoided but may be used in cooking
- Do not use more than twice a week

Bread:
- Unrestricted
- White and whole-meal allowed
- Whole-meal bread is richer in mineral salts, especially po tassium, and it also contains phytic acid, which lowers the amount of calcium absorbed by the intestine
- Fruit loaf (continental, made with oil and not milk) is allowed

Meat:
- Unrestricted
- Ideal: grilled or roasted meat preferred
- Beef, lamb, pork, veal, chicken and turkey are all allowed
- Liver and kidneys are particularly high in sodium and potassium

Small goods:
- These include ham, salami, cabana, pastrami, chicken roll, sausages and liverwurst
- Unrestricted
- Must be included once a day

So, if you can eat a lot of salty meats and you want a son, the boy diet may be manageable for you. For a daughter, it looks like you need to drink lots of milk and consume daily dairy products. If you attempt either of these diets, good luck to you! They don't appear easy to stay on, and although I began a similar one once, I could not keep to it. And again, re-member, consulting a doctor is important both before starting and once on the diet. If anyone in your family has a history of kidney stones or high or low blood pressure, you should probably not attempt a gender diet. And, fortunately, these diets are just temporary; you would not want to stay on them for long. Some experts recommend no longer than three months for the diet. And once you are pregnant, you can start eating normally again—and begin a healthful pregnancy diet!

An Interesting Supplement

Now for one final diet suggestion that I've seen. There is a new diet supplement making the rounds in gender selection discussions: Lydia Pinkham's Herbal Compound. According to In-Gender, a sex selection information website, Lydia Pinkham's Herbal Compound was originally the famous Lydia Pinkham's Vegetable Compound, a patent medicine tonic used to treat "female complaints" and infertility in the Victorian age. A recent (very small) informal survey noted that seven out of eight pregnancies resulted in girl babies when the mother was taking the tonic.

The In-Gender site asks, why does the Lydia Pinkham (LP) make it more likely to conceive a girl? The following ideas have been offered, according to In-Gender:

"• When tested with pH strips, the tonic is quite acidic (a pH of 2). An acidic environment, according to Shettles, is more hostile to sperm and only the hardier female sperm are likely to survive."

"• Black cohosh and other LP ingredients may balance estrogen levels (lower estrogen levels if you are estrogen dominant, or raise it if you are low in estrogen). Some believe that low-estrogen levels make it likely to conceive a girl, and women who are estrogen dominant (higher estrogen levels than progesterone) are more likely to conceive a boy."

In-Gender offers information on how to obtain the Lydia Pinkham compound, suggests how to use it for conception of a baby girl and gives plenty of warnings for consulting a physician first. (See the In-Gender Web address in the appendix.)

The Diet Lowdown

In conclusion, if you are healthy, adventurous and would like to try some inexpensive ways to influence the gender of your next child, a gender diet might be something worth attempting just before trying to conceive. Some people believe in its effectiveness. But, like all of the at-home methods discussed in the previous chapter, there is no guarantee. Nobody can promise you that it will work. Try it if you'll be happy and welcome *any* baby you get, boy or girl (assuming you get pregnant), and maybe you'll have a pleasant surprise.

If you don't think that you can keep to a difficult gender diet, and the Shettles method has not worked for you in your quest for a daughter, you may want to know about still more options. One of them is another, newer timing method for conceiving a daughter that can be tried in the privacy of your home: It's called "O+12." Turn to the next chapter for details.

CHAPTER

4

Out of Australia: O+12

Out of Australia comes the unusual story of a woman who never gave up the dream of a daughter, who kept on having children until her little girl was born, who discovered that there might be yet another way.

Kynzi Rose of Queensland, Australia, conceived her daughter Kristie after six sons and countless Shettles attempts (see chapter 2) over the years. She unexpectedly discovered the way—the method to try one last time—when she was in her doctor's office to discuss a tubal ligation. After six wonderful, much-loved boys, she and her husband found room for one more child, and nine months later her little girl came along … along with a new method for home gender selection. The "O+12" method was born.

Kynzi shares her story. "When we were married in 1975, my husband and I assumed we would have four children and hoped that they would be two boys and two girls. One year and two days after the wedding, our first son was born, and I was as surprised to get a boy first as my husband was pleased." Sixteen months later, another healthy baby boy came along.

"Now for the girls, we thought. A neighbor with two girls came in very excited as she had read an article in a magazine about an American doctor, Landrum Shettles, who had discovered a way to up your chances of choosing the sex of your baby. She wanted a boy next, and we wanted a girl," Kynzi relates. "I read the article, it seemed pretty clear—girls were conceived if you stopped having sex at least three days before ovulation occurred; boys more likely if you waited until ovulation, then had sex. She followed the boy rule, and we followed the girl's. We also had to use a douche before sex, vinegar and water for us. She gave birth to a son, and we gave birth to another son."

After three boys, Kynzi and her husband continued to hope for a daughter. She bought Dr. Shettles' book, *How to Choose the Sex of Your Baby* (see appendix), and religiously followed all of his tips. She also learned how to monitor her ovulation with a basal thermometer chart and with something called TesTape (used by diabetics to test their urine). She read about the suggested gender diets (see chapter 3) and went on a "bland," salt-free diet to try to conceive her daughter. "We were sure we would have a girl and complete the family."

In addition to everything else, Kynzi even tried a new pink "girl" gender gel that a doctor was planning to market. "The instructions were to wait for ovulation and use the gel and have sex just that one night, but we knew better and used it on our cutoff night instead. Pregnancy occurred that month, and we were confident, with all these 'extras,' we would have a girl at last." But it was their fourth son.

Their family was not yet complete. "A friend we hadn't seen for ages came to visit with her newborn baby girl, and it started the old feelings up again. We wanted a baby girl." Kynzi bought the updated version of the Shettles book, and her OB-gynecologist suggested monitoring her monthly ovulation with blood tests and ovary ultrasounds. She adjusted her timing technique further. Another attempt, another boy.

After five great boys, she still was not done. "We could not see where we had gone wrong. We had bought several books on gender selection and all basically agreed with Shettles,"

Kynzi says. "What more could we do?" She learned about the fabled Chinese birth chart (see chapter 2) and they made another baby attempt during a "girl month" according to the chart. She also was on the "dreadful" girl diet again. Another pregnancy, yet another boy.

After six boys, Kynzi's husband said they had to give up. She reluctantly agreed. "I made an appointment to see my OB-gyn for a discussion regarding booking a tubal ligation. When I got there, the doctor had to rush off and do a delivery, so I filled in the time chatting to his receptionist and the clinic nurse. They, of course, found me quite an oddity: a woman with six boys, no girls. The nurse asked if we had ever 'done anything' to influence the gender of our babies, so I related all our attempts to her, and she was quite surprised and mystified where this pre-ovulation idea had sprung from. She pulled a couple of studies done on the gender of babies conceived on certain days of the cycle, and the evidence in these trials showed the opposite to Shettles' ideas: girls were, in fact, coming from having sex *at* ovulation. Babies conceived earlier were far more likely to be boys!" One of these studies was from New Zealand's National Women's Hospital.

"I couldn't believe it," Kynzi continues. "All this time, we had been aiming for the 'boy time,' and the result—boys! I hungrily and regretfully read these charts; I couldn't believe this was happening. There I was ready to give up, and now I knew something different. One chart in particular showed girls only, when the couples chose to abstain until hours after ovulation had occurred.

"I left without seeing the doctor, and went home to think about this new information. Our youngest son was five months old, and my cycle had just returned. In fact, it was day 14, and sure enough, I ovulated that night. I lay there all night, wondering what to do. ..."

A New Method Is Born

Kynzi and her husband decided to "throw caution to the wind" and make one last attempt that day. And although their conception attempt was interrupted when their 5-year-old "burst into the room with an upset stomach," this very fertile couple conceived once again. The next month, they discovered she was pregnant, confirmed by a blood test and ultrasound scan. "I was carrying a baby conceived at 12 hours past ovulation" (thus the abbreviation O+12).

Although a later ultrasound showed there was 60 percent likelihood Kynzi was carrying a girl, she was convinced it was another boy: She says she was still a Shettles believer and the timing of intercourse would indicate a boy; plus the Chinese chart predicted boy for her, and she had given up the girl pre-conception diet.

The baby arrived on Kynzi's due date. "It was indeed a girl! I had to look and check for myself—if this was the mid-wife's idea of a joke, I wasn't laughing. But there she was, a 6-pound, tiny little baby girl," Kynzi says. "Mind you, I still checked at every nappy change—yep, still a girl. I couldn't wait to get her home and dress her up in pink frills, which I did, and I sent everyone a photo of Kristie, pink and frilly from head to toe, in that year's Christmas card. What did I get back? Many friends asking for a naked photo of her—seeing she was definitely our last child, they assumed even a boy would be dressed like that!"

Now that Kynzi was a mother to a baby girl, she "no longer peered into prams containing little pink bundles and wished I had one as well." She says she found herself including "my daughter" in every sentence she uttered for the next few years.

Her four oldest sons are now grown and married and she has a granddaughter. "She, too, is an O+12 baby. I think maybe that's the only way this family will get any girls," Kynzi confides.

"Nowadays there are many high-tech ways of influencing a baby's gender and I am so happy about that—there's no need in having baby after baby just to get one of the chosen gender," she says. "But I consider myself very lucky and blessed to have seven wonderful children and wouldn't change a thing. Even so, I am thankful every day that I achieved my dearest wish, of having a daughter."

So did O+12 timing bring Kynzi her daughter? We may never really know. But as a result of her story, and the studies that appear to corroborate her timing theory, a new method has hit the gender selection grapevine in the past decade.

A few professional studies (typically written about in medical journals) have disproved the Shettles theory of timing, particularly one conducted in Auckland, New Zealand. The "New Zealand Study," as it's commonly called, shows a 2:1 success rate for the occurrence of a male baby being conceived two to four days before ovulation and a female closer to ovulation. This study was carried out to test the accuracy of the Shettles method. The researchers monitored participants to see if Dr. Shettles' timing method proved correct for them. "The results clearly refute the theory that intercourse close to ovulation favors male conceptions," concludes Professor John T. France and others in the journal *Fertility and Sterility* (June 1984, Vol. 41). The only day on which more females than males were conceived in the study was the day *following* ovulation. This was the discovery that Kynzi made.

Many people have been looking beyond Shettles for answers to home sex selection, and some believe they've found it with O+12. In recent years, women around the world have logged onto the Internet and found out about Kynzi and her story, they've passed the information along to others, and many babies have been conceived following her method. Most of those children have been girls.

For couples who are against high-tech sex selection, or cannot afford it, O+12 may be something to consider, although like with the other home methods, there is no guarantee of success. But if you're interested in trying it, this chapter provides instructions for how to follow the method.

O+12, Step by Step

A gender selection practitioner named Maureen has closely followed Kynzi's story and put the details of the O+12 method on her In-Gender website (see appendix). Maureen comments, "The O+12 method advises intercourse about 12 hours *after* ovulation to conceive a girl—contrary to the Shettles method, which predicts a boy will be conceived on the day of ovulation. (Note to boy-seekers: O+12 is a method for attempting to conceive a girl only.)"

In addition to the New Zealand Study, there have been findings showing that the ratio of female-to-male sperm is greater if a man abstains from ejaculation for a period of time before attempting conception. As a result of these combined theories, the O+12 method has been formulated.

Here are instructions for the three main steps of O+12 (obtained from In-Gender):

1. The man must not ejaculate for at least seven days before intercourse (and preferably longer). This doesn't just mean no sex, it means no ejaculation at all. Try to get him to abstain starting from the first day of your cycle. The reason for this is that because female sperm supposedly live longer, an "old" batch of sperm should have more female than male sperm (about 2 percent more, according to some data).

2. Have intercourse only once, 8 to 20 hours *after* ovulation. Start counting the 8 to 20 hours when (a) any *sharp* ovulation pain has subsided (some women get pain in the middle of their cycle indicating ovulation is occurring); (b) your cervical mucus begins to change from an egg-white consistency to creamy or sticky; and/or (c) your cervix begins to become less soft and high. (The mucus consistency and the position of the cervix are both indicators of your stage in the ovulatory cycle.) You should wait to have intercourse until you have seen one high basal body temperature (morning or evening) to confirm that ovulation has truly passed.

3. Do *not* have intercourse again until you are sure you are no longer fertile. Use a condom or wait until you know you're out of the fertile time before having intercourse again, because that "fresh" batch of sperm will be more likely to have more male sperm.

You are past your fertile stage when you have had *three* high temperatures on your basal temperature chart.

Maureen also offers the following comment: "Pinpointing ovulation down to the hour is the key to O+12, and it's not easy. Most ovulation detection methods are just designed to determine the *day* of ovulation, which is generally good enough to achieve (or avoid) pregnancy. For O+12, we have to be ovulation experts."

Additional O+12 Tips

Maureen provides the following tips for O+12:

Tip #1: Practice, practice, practice! Track your ovulation indicators for several practice cycles. Many times, the time of ovulation can only be determined in hindsight. Practice cycles will give you confidence that you know when ovulation is occurring, and they also will give you something to compare with when you're ready to make your attempt.

Tip #2: Use as many ovulation indicators as you can. No matter how regular you are, or how many cycles you practice, each cycle is different. Gather as many clues as you can to determine the real moment of ovulation. Ovulation indicators include basal body temperature, cervical mucus, cervical position, saliva ferning and ovulation prediction kits. The book *Taking Charge of Your Fertility* (see appendix) is a great resource, explaining in detail how to use these methods to determine ovulation.

Tip #3: Watch your cervical mucus and your cervical position. Your cervical mucus usually will change within hours of ovulation, changing from an egg-white consistency to creamy or sticky. Start counting the hours when your mucus has started to change and your cervix is not very high and soft.

Tip #4: Take your basal body temperature effectively. Basal body temperature is a reliable method for detecting that ovulation is truly past, so make sure to take your temps carefully, and wait to have intercourse until you have seen them shift up. However, taking your temps once per day can only tell you that ovulation has occurred within the past 24 hours—and by then you may be too far past ovulation to actually conceive, because the egg only lives about 24 hours.

You also may want to try taking a second temperature in the evening. It will not be as accurate as your morning "at rest" temp, but if you take it at the same time every night after the same routine, you will be able to see a pattern. Taking your temperature twice a day should help you detect ovulation within the past 12 hours. (Note that your body temperature will be different in the evening—you cannot compare your morning and evening temps to each other. You can only compare your morning temps with previous morning temps, and evening temps with previous evening temps.)

Tip #5: Take note of ovulation pain. Ovulation pain, or *mittelschmerz*, can pinpoint the exact time of ovulation—but it also can fool you, because a little random twinge you would have ignored at any other time can mislead you if you're looking for ovulation to occur. Not everyone has this pain, and if you do, it may not be in every cycle.

Some ovulation-pain suggestions:

- Chart any ovulation pain you experience in your practice cycles, and note how it correlates with your other symptoms. You may notice that the pain occurs at about the same time of day that your previous cycle began.
- Recognize the different kinds of pains: a dull achiness before ovulation, a sharp pain at ovulation, crampiness after ovulation.
- The pain should come from toward your side (not from the center) and may be only on one side.

Tip #6: Use ovulation predictor kits as advance warning only. A positive ovulation prediction kit is a sure sign that ovulation is going to occur, but it does *not* give you an accurate prediction of when; it might be anywhere from 12 to 36 hours. When you get your first truly positive predictor, begin watching your *other* ovulation indicators to determine exactly when ovulation is occurring.

On the In-Gender site, Maureen also mentions that you can do O+12 in tandem with the following options: going on a gender diet, taking extra supplements (e.g., calcium, magnesium, cranberry) or douching before intercourse. She suggests a lemon douche made by mixing the fresh-squeezed juice of a half a lemon with an equal part of water, and inserting with the empty bottle from a regular store-bought douche.

Putting O+12 to Use

So there you have it—a new home gender selection method! O+12 is complicated, and it may be more work than some women are willing to do. I considered this method myself at one point (before I conceived my daughter through MicroSort), but I just knew that I was hopeless at figuring out my ovulation time. I never could feel ovulation pains, I balked at the idea of checking cervical mucus and cervix position, and my cycles were too irregular to monitor correctly. Whenever I was ovulating, I didn't have a clue.

However, what is impossible for one woman may be the perfect method for another one. And there are plenty of women who are very good at figuring out what their bodies are doing and making this method something that could work for them.

Victoria of Chicago was one of those. Her sons Nathan, Noah and Nicholas were 10, 4 and 20 months when she attempted the O+12 method for her fourth child. She had tried the Shettles method for her last two pregnancies, using four-day and three-day cutoffs, and had done so for an earlier pregnancy that ended in miscarriage at 12½ weeks. Shettles had not brought her a daughter.

So Victoria was ready for another home method. And she found it on the Internet. "I learned about O+12 from the Gender Determination board at Parent Soup [see appendix]. I read all of Kynzi's e-mails and stories and figured I would be a great candidate," she says. "Everything we did to conceive Nataleigh was exactly the opposite of what we did to conceive our boys, so it made sense to me to try it!

"We were very fortunate to get pregnant our first month trying. Even after having three children, there are no guarantees, and I was 40 years old when I conceived her. I was charting for eight months prior so I knew my cycles very well and was confident that we could time this well for a good

O+12 attempt. Thank goodness, because that diet was awful and would've been the first thing to go if it hadn't worked the first month for us."

The diet Victoria is referring to is the girl diet from the book *The Preconception Gender Diet* (see chapter 3). She was on it for 10 weeks. "I didn't just lower my sodium intake like some have tried but was very strict with the ratio of sodium to calcium, etc. I took calcium plus Vitamin D supplements, along with the magnesium. I also douched with a lemon juice and water mixture before and after BDing [baby dancing—a common euphemism]. I took Sudafed to dry up my cervical mucus and chewed Tums tablets [for the calcium] as well. Most importantly, we included lots of prayer!"

Something in that equation worked, and Victoria came home from the hospital with a baby girl at last.

She reflects on life after a daughter. "Life always changes when you bring a new baby home. Adding a fourth child to our family wasn't much harder. I won't say that having a daughter has changed 'life' for me, but everything about having a girl is different from having boys and I'm thoroughly enjoying the experience of raising both genders. We get lots of comments when we're out with the entire family. Four kids get a lot of attention regardless of gender," she laughs. "Most people just have to say something like, 'Oh, you finally got your girl after three boys!'

"I suppose the one thing that has changed for me is how much I enjoy shopping for girlie clothing and accessories and how much *she* enjoys it as well. I love to buy for my boys as well, but it just isn't the same."

Victoria, like O+12 pioneer Kynzi, ultimately got a happy ending to her gender quest. It is not definite that O+12 can be credited for that, but this method certainly has spawned a new way of looking at timing for gender conception.

Low-Tech Vs. High-Tech

For some women, home methods are as far as they want to go to try to reach their gender dream. Gender selection is definitely an ethical issue for some, and many are not willing to "tamper with nature" any further than timing intercourse at home. Thus, the O+12 method, like the Shettles method before it, may be something worth trying.

But if you have tried a low-tech method and it didn't work, or you want more of a guarantee or a "sure thing," then you may want to look beyond these methods. For me, home methods were not successful. I was willing to look outside for an answer. The following chapters will discuss the latest in high-tech gender selection.

CHAPTER

5

The Spinning of Sperm

Before there was "Microsorting," there was sperm "spinning." Probably the oldest of the high-tech methods, sperm spinning is done in several labs around the United States (and across the world), with the purpose of dividing male sperm from female sperm before insemination. Using this technique, a couple can increase their chances of having a baby of the sex of their choice, although, like with low-tech methods, there is no guarantee.

In the early 1980s, Dr. Ronald J. Ericsson of Gametrics Limited developed what he calls the Ericsson Albumin Method, a technique that attempts to separate the girl and boy chromosomes by filtering patients' sperm through a water-soluble protein solution called albumin. Another procedure separates sperm through a centrifuge. Because Y-chromosome-bearing sperm (for males) are lighter, they supposedly rise to the top; and the heavier, denser X-chromosome-bearing sperm (for females) are said to sink to the bottom. Doctors then perform artificial insemination during a woman's anticipated ovulation time using the separated, enriched sperm according to the gender that couples request. Requests for girls appear to be higher than for boys (a common occurrence with high-tech gender selection in the United States).

The Ericsson mission is "to provide safe, reliable and proven technology to allow parents to select the sex of their child." The providers claim a success rate of 78 to 85 percent for male babies, and a rate of 73 to 75 percent for females.

Ericsson Basics

Couples who decided to undergo a sex selection procedure provide a fresh semen sample to an Ericsson-licensed laboratory for processing. This often is scheduled three to four hours before the insemination, on a day that is the woman's most likely ovulation time. Sometimes there are two separate inseminations performed (depending on a few factors).

"The insemination requires only several minutes," explains Dr. Ronald Ericsson. "The important factors are fresh semen of good quality and a known time for ovulation." A woman's monthly ovulation is monitored using her past menstrual patterns, her basal body temperature charts (see chapters 2 and 4), physical examinations and hormone tests.

The typical time it takes for an average woman to get pregnant using the Ericsson technology and artificial insemination is three attempts; sometimes it takes less, sometimes more. But there is no guarantee of pregnancy.

"Human reproduction is not a very efficient process, as evidenced by the fact that only about 20 percent of couples trying to conceive naturally do so in any given month," according to company information provided to prospective sex selection participants. And if a couple conceives after the Ericsson procedure, "The outcome of pregnancies so conceived can never be guaranteed, because sperm isolation does not completely separate X from Y chromosome-bearing sperm. The statistics for each procedure will be discussed with you before proceeding."

The Ericsson method is a patented technique, licensed to 48 fertility centers around the country and the world. States with locations include California, Connecticut, Florida, Maine, Michigan, Montana, New Mexico, New York, Texas and Washington; internationally, there are centers in East Asia, Hong Kong, India, Israel, Jordan, Macau, Malaysia, the Netherlands, Pakistan, Panama, South America and the United Kingdom. (For contact information, see the appendix for Dr. Ericsson's Gametrics website.) Thousands of babies have been born through the Ericsson method.

Going for the Boy

Mona of New Hampshire has one of those children. She and her husband, Jeff, had two daughters and were always hoping to have four children—two boys and two girls. Mona knew that her chances of having a third girl were high, so she started "surfing the Web" to find ways to up their odds of a boy for the family. "We both wanted a son," she says.

Mona learned about timing intercourse and using douches to change the acidity of the vaginal tract, both home methods to influence gender (discussed in chapter 2), but then she stumbled upon the idea of the Ericsson Albumin Method. She knew she had found something that might substantially increase their odds of conceiving a baby boy.

So she went for it. But first she had to convince Jeff. "He was skeptical at first. I did all of the research." She printed out information from the Internet and laid it all out for him.

After he agreed to try the Ericsson method of sperm separation, they made their first attempt, driving three hours to the closest sex selection clinic to do it. It was a simple artificial insemination procedure, done just once. But there was no pregnancy. Another month they tried again, and this second time they succeeded.

"It was an absolutely wonderful experience," Mona comments. "I highly recommend it."

She says she took no medications other than folic acid and prenatal vitamins, starting three months before they wanted to get pregnant. One insemination cycle cost them "less than $1,000" for everything.

"I thought it was very reasonable," she says. They spent a total of about $1,500 for the two cycles together—"and I got a boy." She feels this is a great value for the money, must less expensive than other gender selection technologies.

"I'm really so, so thrilled with my baby boy," Mona says. At 1 year old now, he is walking and is very healthy. And she enjoys having children of both genders. "He is just so different from my two girls." (The girls are now 7 and 3.)

Mona and Jeff have only told a handful of people how their little boy was conceived—her sister, Jeff's parents and a couple of friends. They are not sure how other people would react.

And what about that fourth child? Mona says they may try to have one more baby, and they'll definitely consider going back to the Ericsson sex selection center, so their son can have a brother like his two sisters have each other.

Facts About Ericsson

Mona's experience with the Ericsson method is typical of the average attempt, including the costs they paid. The technology is not prohibitively expensive. "The cost varies by location within the USA or international sperm centers," says Dr. Ericsson. "The range in cost is from $600 to $1,200 per try." This is less than half the price of a similar insemination attempt with MicroSort.

The Ericsson procedures have been done for more than 25 years with no known health problems to child or mother. The likelihood of miscarriage is reportedly the same as in the general population, as are the chances of any birth defects. The technology is open to most couples who want to try gender preselection, although they should first attend a consultation, a medical history must be provided, and the woman must undergo a gynecological exam before starting.

"Couples who use sex selection are almost always parents and they are seeking the sex of a child they do not have," according to Dr. Ericsson. "The average number of children is slightly more than two, and these children are almost always the sex opposite of what the couple is seeking. Those who want a girl have boys and those who have girls want a boy. And, they want it for the last child. Sex selection is definitely a form of family planning."

There are, however, some couples who come to an Ericsson clinic for a purpose other than simple family planning. These are people who need to conceive a child of a particular gender for medical reasons—because of a sex-linked (or, X-linked) disorder that is carried down through the family tree. Dr. Ericsson admits that the percentage of couples who come for this reason is small, for a few different reasons.

"Most sex-linked diseases affect the male with the mother as the carrier of the gene. This means if the child is male, it has a 1 out of 2 chance of having the disease. As these sex-linked diseases are either life-threatening or lifelong-debilitating, most couples need to give serious thought to having a child," Dr. Ericsson explains. "There is no method that gives a 100 percent probability that a sex-selected child will be female—other than sexing an embryo prior to implantation." (For details on embryo gender selection, see chapter 9.)

"Also, the use of sex selection has not been available long enough to the public for this technology to become commonplace. The percentage of couples who use sex selection for sex-linked diseases will certainly increase in the future," Dr. Ericsson predicts.

Building a Healthy Family

One couple who did come to a gender preselection clinic for such purposes are Elizabeth and Kent of Maine.

"Ever since I can remember, Duchenne's muscular dystrophy has affected my life," Elizabeth explains. "My brother William was diagnosed at age 6 and his physical strength deteriorated until his passing at the age of 20. I have seen his frustration, fear and struggle firsthand, and it wasn't easy to watch someone you love hurt so."

She continues, "I am a confirmed carrier of DMD, a sex-linked genetic disease, and this has affected family planning for my husband and I. As long as we have been sexually active, we have always had to be careful not to have an unplanned pregnancy. We have not wanted to risk the conception of a male child, as there is naturally a 50/50 chance.

"Basically, my husband and I have wanted to avoid having a male child if at all possible. When we finally decided to start our family, we knew there may be a way for us to choose the gender of our baby. It had been in the media/news."

Elizabeth, who lives in Lewiston, Maine, learned about Dr. Michael T. Drouin, a physician with a practice in Lewiston that covers the treatment of male infertility and gender preselection. (See appendix for contact information.)

"When it was time for me to see a gynecologist for the first time, my mom recommended Dr. Drouin to me because she had heard that he was doing different things with fertility and such," Elizabeth explains. "It was years later at our first family planning consultation with him that we learned about the Ericsson method. It would bring our 50/50 chance for conceiving a girl up to almost 80/20."

Elizabeth and Kent went ahead with the Ericsson procedure at Women's Health Center in Lewiston and conceived a baby after four attempts. Elizabeth used the fertility medication

Clomid (medical name, clomiphene citrate), as was recommended.

Their journey to build their family was not an easy one, but they continued on it. "We braved through the clomiphene mood swings and abstinence, as well as the injections and the insemination. We didn't mind much because we wanted a healthy child, and were doing what we had to do. It was a little frustrating when we didn't get pregnant until the fourth try for our firstborn child, but we persevered. The end result was worth the effort, and the experience overall was positive. It was the time between conception and the amniocentesis that was the worst unnerving, to say the least." But Elizabeth was carrying a healthy little girl.

After their daughter was born, they eventually planned their attempt for a sister for her. This time, they looked in a different direction—MicroSort, where patients with sex-linked genetic issues were given three free cycles (see chapter 6).

"In trying to get pregnant with our second child, we were involved in the MicroSort study through the Genetics & IVF Institute," explains Elizabeth. "Louise at Dr. Drouin's office steered us this way because the success rate for female gender was 95 percent. We were so excited about the percentage that we packed our bags for Virginia—three times. The staff there was wonderful, and we did some sightseeing. However, after our three study-funded attempts failed, we decided to try the Ericsson method at home again. It would have been much more comforting during the time between conception and the amniocentesis to know that you had a 95/5 ratio, but to continue with MicroSort would have been too costly."

They conceived their second daughter after only one try. They have the Women's Health Center to thank for it. "Dr. Drouin, Louise and the staff took good care of my husband and I, and we would recommend their talents to folks such as ourselves," says Elizabeth.

"We have our happy, healthy family."

Opinions on Ericsson Method

Elizabeth and Kent had a happy ending to their gender quest, as did Mona and Jeff, but not everyone has been so confident about the accuracy of the Ericsson Albumin Method.

After some controversy arose in the 1990s over the effectiveness of the human serum albumin (HSA) method of separating X and Y sperm, two researchers from the Gender Choice Centre in Hong Kong tested the procedure. G.A. Rose and A. Wong applied the HSA separation method using the technique as described by Dr. Ericsson and others in a *Nature* article (1973, Vol. 246). The separated specimen was examined for X- and Y-bearing spermatozoa by fluorescent in-situ using appropriate DNA probes.

"Of 18 couples wanting boys, 13 had single boys, one had twin boys, and one had twins comprising one boy and one girl," according to Rose and Wong in *Human Reproduction* (1998, Vol. 13). "Only three single girls were born. This success rate of 83 percent is significantly different from the usual expected ratio."

Parenthood.com, a parenting website, has taken a look at gender selection and the Ericsson method and noted the timing of artificial insemination with Ericsson, which takes place at ovulation. "Based on Dr. Shettles' theory of timed intercourse, one would expect more males with this method due to the timing, regardless of whether or not the separation actually worked, and this is what has been found consistently," Parenthood.com comments. "Interestingly, when the sperm samples were studied after the separation, they still seemed to be 50/50 X and Y."

Parenthood.com refers to the *Human Reproduction* article written by the Hong Kong researchers and notes that they performed careful DNA studies on the supposed X-rich and

Y-rich fractions produced by the separation. The researchers stated that examination of the enriched sperm samples "showed no change in the normal and equal numbers of X- and Y-bearing spermatozoa after the HSA separation procedure." In other words, the ratio of boy sperm to girl sperm was still 50/50.

"However, the birth data told a different story!" comments Parenthood. "Out of 18 couples wanting boys, 13 delivered single boys and one had twin boys! This gave an 83 success rate for this method. They concluded that the Ericsson method did enhance the odds for a male child, but not by the previously thought mechanism. Maybe Dr. Shettles was right!"

The Hong Kong researchers have another take on it: "It is tentatively proposed that passage through the HSA inactivates X-bearing spermatozoa more than Y-bearing spermatozoa, even though this is not apparent simply on inspection of sperm motility," wrote Rose and Wong.

So whatever the reason, the Ericsson Albumin Method appears to work for achieving male babies—a fact that may be confirmed by its worldwide clinic rates. Couples who want boys usually are satisfied. Those seeking girls, however, have not been as successful.

Not So Good for Girls?

In an informal survey I've done over the years of women who have tried the Ericsson method at least once for a baby girl, of those who got pregnant (and some did not), as many seemed to conceive boys as produced girls. Unfortunately, the method may not be the answer to high-tech gender selection for female babies.

The *New York Times* recently ran a story in its Sunday magazine about a woman (Mara Silverman) who, after "three amazing, healthy boys," decided with her husband to do sperm spinning to try to preselect a baby girl. They conceived on their first attempt and ended up with twins. During the pregnancy they found out the genders. Both were boys.

For the Silvermans, like other couples trying for a female baby, sperm spinning was obviously ineffective.

Dr. Peter Liu, co-founder of the London Gender Clinic in the United Kingdom, has worked with a variety of sex selection technologies, including the Ericsson Albumin Method. "We must point out that not all the sperm centers licensed to use the albumin sperm separation method choose to use this treatment for selecting girls," he comments on his sex selection website. "Our experience with this treatment for female sex selection is that the results can be rather variable and unpredictable, which makes it difficult for us to endorse its use. This is not to say we are disputing the claims of the doctors using this method for selecting girls, but in our hands we were not entirely satisfied with the results of the procedure."

Another gender selection physician, Dr. Frank Comhaire of Gent University Hospital, Belgium, states, "Perhaps the Ericsson method (using an albumin gradient) is reasonably accurate for Y-bearing spermatozoa (sons). However, there are few statistics on this method."

Several medical professionals have dismissed the albumin technique as being very effective, and for female babies, most believe that the success rate is 70 percent at most.

The American Society for Reproductive Medicine comments on this method and similar sex selection techniques: "Many methods of preconception gender selection through sperm separation have been tried, such as albumin gradients, Percoll gradients, Sephadex columns and a modified swim-up technique. None has shown consistent X- and Y-sperm cell separation or validated success in producing offspring of the desired gender." The organization made this conclusion in the journal *Fertility and Sterility* (2001, Vol. 75, No. 5).

Although the 70 percent accuracy rate of girl sex selection with the Ericsson method may not be the best-odds scenario, it is still better than nature's option of 50/50 (or even lower than 50 percent, in some couples' history). So a variety of couples, armed with this information and realizing their chances, continue to go to the numerous Ericsson clinics and attempt to make a girl baby.

The Benefit of Clomid

One thing that can help is the use of Clomid in a female sex selection cycle. Clomid causes the hormonal induction of ovulation for women who take the oral prescription medication at the beginning of their monthly cycle. Studies have shown that the combination of using Clomid and performing albumin separation of sperm—in conjunction with artificial insemination—has increased the odds of producing a female baby. As a result, when patients come to an Ericsson clinic seeking a daughter, the staff will recommend that the woman use Clomid for her planned cycle.

"There are a number of papers in the scientific literature that provide evidence that the hormonal induction of ovulation will skew the sex ratio from the normal majority of males to a majority of females," Dr. Ericsson confirms. "The reason for this shift in the sex ratio remains unexplained. We use the drug clomiphene citrate as part of the protocol for female selection. It cannot be used for male selection as this would negate the increase for males. We learned through clinical trials that the use of clomiphene citrate in conjunction with sperm isolation will increase the percent of females by 25 percent."

In surveys I've seen that detail the results both of natural conceptions as well as those produced by artificial insemination, there does seem to be an increase in female babies when the woman has used Clomid prior to or during the conception cycle.

Ericsson or MicroSort?

In conclusion, if you decide to go to an Ericsson sex selection clinic—or another clinic that performs something
similar to spinning for sperm separation—your odds will be
better if you're trying for a little boy. If you are looking for a
little girl, you take your chances. If you do decide to try the
Ericsson Albumin Method (and there are clinics and the main
company listed in the appendix) and undergo the girl sex selection procedure, remember that Clomid may increase your
chance of success.

While the Ericsson method has less expensive fees, better
pregnancy rates and, currently, more locations than MicroSort,
it appears not to have the gender success rates that the new
technology has. Elizabeth's story notwithstanding, there are
not as many gender success stories that I have found for
people who have attempted sperm spinning as there are for
MicroSort—especially if one is seeking a daughter.

For the odds of 90 percent or higher for a baby girl,
MicroSort appears to be the best bet for reaching that gender
goal. For me, there was no other choice. MicroSort was in my
area (Ericsson is not), and, if I could get pregnant, it appeared
to be closest to a sure thing for me.

I wasn't yet willing to give up my journey for a daughter.
If you're still looking for your answer, read the next couple of
chapters to learn about MicroSort.

CHAPTER

6

The MicroSort Way

The drive to reach a goal—the determination to see a long-time dream come true—can be a very strong thing. It can occupy your everyday thoughts, it can shape your daily activities, it can become an obsession. It can make you do things you never imagined doing.

That is what happened to me when I decided I wanted a daughter. And even as the months and years went by and it did not occur, and I gave birth to two wonderful, priceless little boys, my longing did not go away. In some ways, it became stronger. I didn't want to be just a "boy mom"—I really wanted to experience raising children of both genders. And because I did not want to fail in my journey, and I needed all of my efforts to mean something, I just could not give up. I continued to carry that image in my head of a little girl posing for a photo, flanked by her two big brothers.

Why else would someone end up in the small consulting room of a nondescript building of an infertility clinic in Fairfax, Va., especially someone with no known fertility problems, speaking to strangers about the desire for a daughter? What could drive someone to subject herself to regular blood draws and pelvic ultrasounds, to clinicians poking around and checking her egg follicle sizes and the thickness of her uterine lining, to monitoring and reporting her sexual intercourse days—not to mention having to ask her husband to provide a sample of that most private of things, his semen, for a sperm count?

Only a fixation that won't go away could push someone to do this. And for me, MicroSort was the answer to the unending question that seemed to rule my days: How could I make my dream finally come true? How can I conceive a daughter when it looked like my husband and I could only make boys? Everything I had been hoping for during the past few years had led me to this place. And nothing behind those doors would make me turn away once I got there.

MicroSort Basics

So here are the facts about MicroSort. The staff at the Genetics & IVF Institute (GIVF) in Fairfax help participants choose the sex of their baby through flow cytometry, a procedure in which DNA is stained with a fluorescent dye and sorted. Instead of comparing the swimming ability of the sperm, MicroSort compares their size. This technology capitalizes on the fact that X-chromosome sperm (which produce girls) have 2.8 percent more genetic material than Y-chromosome sperm (which produce boys). So the female sperm appear slightly larger than the male sperm. In addition, when a florescent dye is applied to the sperm, the females glow more brightly than the males. Working with an expensive MicroSort machine, technicians use the cytometer to distinguish these differences in brightness and divvy up the sperm as they move through the machine one at a time. The sperm are washed, and the sorted, enriched specimen is put into a type of ice chest for the subsequent insemination or fertilization process.

MicroSort, whose research began in 1991, is currently in clinical trials. Couples who would like to be candidates for the study must meet the following qualifications: They must be married, they must test negative for HIV and Hepatitis, they should have no history of serious birth defects, the woman must be under 40, and they must be trying for a gender that is the least represented in the family. In other words, if they have one of each gender, they don't qualify for the clinical trial; but someone like us, who had two boys and no girl at the time, were good candidates. This is known as sorting for family balancing. The clinic also will do the sort procedure for couples who carry X-linked genetic diseases (such as hemophilia and Duchenne's muscular dystrophy), regardless of the genders in their family. Such couples have been able to get financial help from MicroSort for their conception attempts.

To date, the clinic reports more than 500 pregnancies so far after the use of MicroSort; 419 babies have been born (as of this book's press time), with more due to be delivered.

"We plan to evaluate 750 babies through the first year of life prior to submitting our request for approval to the FDA for the family balancing indication," says Dr. Keith Blauer, MicroSort clinical director. "We anticipate that the 750 pregnancies will be achieved in 2006, but the final review will probably not be completed until 2007."

Dr. Blauer joined GIVF in 1997, and "I became actively involved in the clinical management of MicroSort patients in 1998. I became the primary investigator in 2000."

GIVF investigations have shown that 85 percent of couples who have participated in MicroSort's clinical trials did so for family balancing purposes, and a majority of them were looking for daughters.

Conception with MicroSort

There are two methods of trying to achieve pregnancy with MicroSort: intrauterine insemination (IUI) or in-vitro fertilization (IVF). This chapter explains IUI, the easier, more common and less expensive method. (See the next couple of chapters for information on IVF.)

The IUIs must be performed in the MicroSort center, not at an outside clinic. This is due to the fact that after the sperm sample has been sorted in the Fairfax laboratory, and then frozen for delivery, there will be a much reduced number of motile sperm after thawing, not nearly enough total motile sperm to achieve adequate pregnancy rates with IUI. ("Motile," like "mobile," means that the sperm are capable of movement.) MicroSort's data show that fewer than 3 percent of women will conceive after an IUI using sorted, frozen sperm. For that reason, all IUIs must be done in Fairfax, unless patients (namely on the West Coast) choose to go to the new MicroSort location at the Huntington Reproductive Center in Laguna Hills, Calif. Either way, the staff performing the IUI on the prospective mother must be working with fresh, recently sorted sperm—at one of the two current locations.

There are no guarantees with MicroSort. First, pregnancy is not a given. In fact, it can be rather difficult, especially if doing an IUI: The MicroSort clinic average cumulative pregnancy rate (at the time of this book's publication) is 16.6 percent per treatment cycle. It may take several cycles to get pregnant, if at all. Even if a woman has been very fertile before becoming a MicroSort participant, that does not mean she will conceive. The average sperm numbers, after the sort and wash process, are about 200,000 sperm, a low number for achieving pregnancy through artificial insemination. At the present time, those are the numbers they are getting for the process; hopefully the reality will get better.

Sometimes injectible fertility drugs are used to increase the chance of success. Most women who attempt a MicroSort IUI use the oral fertility drug Clomid, which helps guarantee that they will produce one or two egg follicles for the insemination. But to help push this process along even more, some participants will use injectible follicle-stimulating hormones (FSH), such as Gonal-F, Follistim or Repronex, which can help produce multiple follicles. This practice also increases the odds of multiple babies if a pregnancy occurs; twins or triplets are a very real possibility. Usually MicroSort will not recommend injectible medication unless a woman has already tried at least one Clomid cycle and did not respond well to the drug and/or could not get pregnant.

Some trial participants may attempt a "natural" MicroSort IUI, meaning using no medications at all to help with follicle growth. Pregnancy odds are usually not as good with a natural cycle as they are with a Clomid one, but it can be done.

Another non-guarantee of MicroSort is the gender—although this has much better success than its pregnancy rates. MicroSort results show that for couples sorting for a girl, 91 percent of their pregnancies are female, and couples sorting for boys have a 76 percent likelihood of a male pregnancy. So, occasionally, despite all efforts otherwise, an "opposite" conception may happen, though this is rare, especially for girls. As MicroSort puts it, "A child of the desired gender cannot be guaranteed because the current technology does not completely exclude either female or male sperm cells from the enriched sample." The enriched sample is "the resulting portion of the semen specimen after MicroSort sperm separation that contains an increased number of sperm cells of the desired gender."

So there is always a slight chance that a woman may get pregnant from the small amount of the "other" gender sperm that get into the sorted, enriched specimen. After the husband makes his donation and it is sorted, technicians follow a laboratory procedure using DNA analysis to examine the resulting specimen, and participants may be told their sort "purity"— the percentage of X or Y sperm. For example, if a couple trying for a girl ends up with a 93 percent purity, that means that 93 percent of the sample planned for the insemination will include X-bearing sperm and just 7 percent will include Y-bearing sperm. For boy sorts, the purity is usually lower than

90 percent. The sorting technology currently is more effective for obtaining X-bearing sperm.

Finding Success

Most couples who go to MicroSort and are fortunate enough to get pregnant, and stay pregnant, end up eventually bringing home a baby of the gender sought. So far, MicroSort's success record appears to be unprecedented for any form of preconception gender selection.

None of the other methods discussed previously in this book is as promising as MicroSort for selecting a child's gender. Many doctors feel that the other options provide no more than a 50/50 chance, the same as nature allows.

"The success rates for these other methods are not good," Dr. Larry Lipshultz, a Baylor College of Medicine professor of urology, told the *Los Angeles Times* when MicroSort opened up its laboratory in the L.A. area. "They are very comparable to flipping a coin."

But MicroSort lets you choose which side of the coin will come up. And that's what I did.

The Start of My Journey

My own MicroSort journey was a long one and though ultimately successful, it did not start out that way. It began in the fall of 2000, when my second son was a little over 1. Luckily, my husband was amenable to having a third child, though we had earlier talked about having only two. He was basically supportive of my "obsession" for a daughter and agreed to give MicroSort a shot. So we came up with the money and started our first IUI. At the time, it cost $2,500 per cycle. (As of press time, the prices range from $2,550 to $3,950, depending on which options you choose, such as outside monitoring or MicroSort monitoring, and whether or not you choose an FSH medicated cycle.) At the time, that price tag included full clinical monitoring (with ultrasounds and bloodwork), the sperm sort and the insemination.

Before starting the cycle, we filled out an application with our medical and family histories, we had an in-person consultation with a nurse-clinician who went over our paperwork and answered our questions (this can be done over the phone if you do not live convenient to the clinic), we both had bloodwork done to rule out any infectious diseases, and my husband had to provide a semen analysis. If the prospective father does not have good sperm count and motility, a MicroSort IUI will be a waste of time and money, because the specimen that he will provide for sorting will be drastically reduced by the time it gets to the IUI. Men who don't have a minimum sperm count and motility in the semen analysis are recommended to repeat the analysis or to forgo doing an IUI. And when couples *are* accepted into the program, they are recommended to have a certain period of abstinence before the IUI day so that the sperm donated for the sorting and insemination will be of the best possible quality.

Luckily, my husband's semen analysis results were satis-factory and we began the process for our first cycle. We had chosen to do a Clomid cycle, and I was instructed to take one tablet per day for five days near the beginning of my cycle (day 1 starts the first day of the menstrual period). I had no side effects from Clomid, though this is not the case for many women. Then I began regular monitoring. I drove to the clinic every few days, signed myself in and proceeded to have my blood drawn (to check my levels of estrogen and luteinizing hormone) and my uterus and ovaries "scanned." This moni-toring gives us an idea of when ovulation may occur. The painless scans showed, upon an ultrasound screen, the number and size of any egg follicles I might have ripening as a result of the Clomid I had taken. I had two growing. My uterine lining also was measured; it usually needs to be a certain thickness for embryo implantation to be successful.

The staff at MicroSort usually were very warm, forthcoming and knowledgeable. In my experiences at their offices, I always dealt with the nurse-clinicians, women who seemed to know what they were doing and were enthusiastic about making this "experiment" succeed. I was there during the first years of the trial, and it was exciting (though a little scary) to be part of the new technology.

My first IUI was getting close. When my egg follicles became a certain size (reaching maturity) and my hormones reached a certain level, it was time for a shot of human chorionic gonadotropin (hCG), an injection that would release the eggs from their follicles within a certain time period and help properly time the moment of insemination. All patients, whether they do a natural cycle, choose a Clomid cycle or go with injectible hormones, are advised to have this hCG shot. We were given an instruction sheet for what time and how to do the injection, and my husband was in charge of giving it to me, in the hip/buttock area. I was nervous, but fortunately he was able to carry it off and give me the shot correctly!

My First Insemination

Ovulation, or the releasing of the eggs from their ovary follicles into the fallopian tubes, is expected to take place approximately 36 hours after the hCG injection. I had my shot at about 10 p.m. one day, and a day and a half later I was supposed to report to the clinic for my insemination. On that day, my husband drove to the clinic early in the morning to provide his "donation," which he produced in a room designated for that activity (complete with magazines to help the men along). Some couples, especially if they are staying at a hotel right near the clinic, choose to produce the semen specimen in a private room and drive the provided container with its contents immediately over to the lab. We lived a little far away for that, and I wanted to make sure the semen specimen stayed intact, so my husband produced it at the clinic.

When he was done, he handed over his container to a lab technician. The container was immediately labeled with our last name and the gender we were trying for (X). Most couples there are trying for a girl. And I have never heard of any mixups whatsoever with the lab specimens.

My husband's sperm then spent much of the day going through the MicroSort machine, getting sorted, while I waited anxiously for the results and for my IUI later that day. Our resulting sorted specimen, which ended up with a purity of about 90 percent, was put in an ice chest with its identity (husband's name and "X-sort") clearly marked on the test tube. Then it was time for the insemination.

When I arrived around 4 p.m., nervous but excited, I was brought back to one of the same examining rooms where earlier in the week I had had my monitoring. The nurse-clinicians did the whole process. First, I was given another pelvic ultrasound scan to check whether my egg follicles had erupted yet or were starting to erupt, releasing the eggs. My husband and I got to see all of this on the ultrasound screen. Then I was shown the labeled test tube of sperm to verify its accuracy (a step that gave me some reassurance as I lay there on the examining bed), and the procedure began.

The insemination felt similar to a pelvic exam, with the benefit of getting to watch everything on the screen: we saw the catheter of sperm placed in my uterus, where the clinician pushed the plunger and released the little swimmers. We watched, hoping those little female sperm would find an egg and do their job!

After the IUI, I was instructed to lie flat on my back for at least 20 minutes, before going home and starting the countdown to pregnancy testing about two weeks later. I started with home pregnancy tests, never wanting to see a dark line more in my life, and then I came in to the clinic for a scheduled blood beta hCG test, which would confirm any news.

Unfortunately, although I had faint lines on my first home tests, they soon disappeared with subsequent testing (I did a lot of them!), and my blood test at MicroSort showed evidence of a "chemical pregnancy." This meant that my hCG number was so low that it looked like I might have experienced a fertilization between egg and sperm, but implantation failed to occur. The very early pregnancy did not continue. This is in effect a very early miscarriage, and apparently it is quite common although the majority of women who experience a chemical pregnancy never realize that it has happened. I only found out because of my obsessive early testing and then the clinical blood test.

This first "almost" success at MicroSort encouraged me that it might be possible to get pregnant there, and I was determined to keep on trying. I had heard about people who had had it happen. I had "met" other women through the Internet who had tried MicroSort or were considering it. Karen of New York was one of the lucky ones; a year earlier she had gotten pregnant her first try doing an unmedicated IUI. She shared her experiences with me and encouraged me not to give up, especially since I lived so close to MicroSort's headquarters in Virginia.

Karen's Story

Karen had originally gotten her inspiration from, of all things, daytime television. At that time, she and her husband had three little boys, having had tried Shettles timing for a girl in their last pregnancy. They were still hoping for a daughter. "In March 1999, I was watching the Oprah show on medical miracles and out comes a woman with a couple of boys who did gender selection to have a girl," Karen explains. "Right away I ran to my computer to look up all the information I could about MicroSort, and by the time my husband came home for dinner I had everything printed out on the kitchen table. We had always wanted four kids and now since there was a way to sway the odds in favor of a girl, we were going for it!"

Karen went to her local obstetrician's office for monitoring of her ovulatory cycle, an option for people who live outside of MicroSort's Northern Virginia area. The first month they were going to MicroSort, she ovulated too early and "missed my chance." They tried again two months later. On the day she turned 29 in November 1999, she reported to her doctor's office for her first day of monitoring for her MicroSort IUI. Her doctor told her that she was ready to go, and she left for Fairfax, Va., that night. Her sons were then 6, 4 and 2.

"We decided to collect the sample at the hotel and bring it to MicroSort. His sperm count was 541 million before the sort, 314,000 after the sort, with 88 percent purity for X-sperm. My uterine lining was 11 [a thick measurement perfect for implantation] at the time of the IUI. I had the hCG shot about 42 hours prior to the IUI. The egg already was released by the time the IUI was done."

Karen got pregnant, and in July 2000, her daughter Meghan was born and her family was transformed. "At first, having a girl was just like having another baby—no-sleep nights," she laughs. "And it was tough with four kids under 7 years old. Meghan is now 3 years old and such a princess. I see her father and brothers let her get away with everything. They all dote on her. I don't know if it's because she is the baby of the family or because she is a girl.

"I love that she has older brothers that are so protective of her. Now that she is older and can talk, she is such a girl—always asking when we can go shopping and when can she get her nails done!"

Karen reflects on the changes in her life. "I see our relationship is different already. Not because I love her any more than the boys; it's just different from the boys. I feel like I will be not only her mother but her best friend.

"I always wanted people to know that I am just your ordinary suburban soccer mom, who tried to change the odds to have a girl, so I can enjoy the trials and tribulations that come with raising both genders."

My Journey, To Be Continued

Karen was lucky; she got pregnant her first actual try, and she did not have to use any fertility medications. But as my own experience shows—and certainly many others—there is no guarantee of pregnancy at MicroSort, and the IUI success rate is not that high yet.

And although I personally did everything I could think of to increase my pregnancy chances—including following fertility tips and eventually trying the injectible fertility drug Gonal-F—I never was able to get a baby from an IUI. Although I knew of other women, like Karen, who had succeeded, I was not able to. After my first MicroSort IUI attempt, I went on to experience one more chemical pregnancy and some other failed IUIs. It was time for me to stop trying this avenue.

Please read on to learn what finally brought us—and other couples—a daughter.

CHAPTER

7

IVF: Better Pregnancy Odds

From the early days of the first "test tube baby"—in 1978, when Louise Brown was born in Oldham, England, to a media frenzy—in-vitro fertilization (IVF) has been fascinating the general public as we've seen what modern medicine can do and we've realized that conception could occur in a laboratory, rather than just inside the female body.

IVF is no longer a rarity in our communities—it's common in fertility clinics throughout the world. Australia, France and Israel all have been strong on the IVF clinic front; and by 1988, the United States reportedly had more than 160 clinics. The first U.S. baby conceived in a laboratory, Elizabeth Jordan Carr, was born in 1981. Her parents used the Jones Institute in Norfolk, Va. Today, many people know someone who has done IVF. And every year there seems to be more to learn in the field of reproductive endocrinology and embryology, with new strides continually being made.

IVF has miraculously solved the problem of many types of infertility—and it has made parents out of many people who may never have had a biological child otherwise.

IVF also brought me my daughter, born in July 2002. For me, what this science did was amazing, because it put together my eggs and my husband's MicroSorted sperm, and it gave us a great opportunity to make a little girl.

For those couples who are unable to achieve pregnancy with the combination of MicroSort and artificial insemination (which can be difficult, because of the reduced sperm numbers), or for those with an infertility issue, IVF is the way to go to be successful with MicroSort. The overall IVF clinical pregnancy rate is higher than that of an intrauterine insemination (IUI) with MicroSort; it's about 33 percent per cycle (which includes IVF procedures done by MicroSort collaborators in other clinics).

What's Involved in IVF

The standard IVF process involves several steps, beginning with ovarian stimulation to produce several mature eggs that can be harvested from the ovaries before they are released from their follicles. Then the woman's mature eggs are aspirated from her ovaries through a needle (in what is often called "egg retrieval") in an outpatient clinical procedure, and they are placed in a special medium for a few hours, followed by her husband's processed sperm being added to the culture dish with the eggs. If fertilization and cell division succeed, some of the resulting embryos are put back into the prospective mother's uterus (in what is called "embryo transfer") a few days after the retrieval. To become a baby, the embryo must then successfully implant in the lining of the uterus.

In a natural ovulatory cycle, woman usually only release one egg per month. But with IVF there often is a high attrition rate with the retrieved eggs, so producing more eggs increases the chances of a cycle's success. Most clinics have their IVF patients inject daily follicle-stimulating hormone drugs to cause multiple ovulation, or lots of eggs. It is not uncommon for a fertile woman to produce 15 to 20 egg follicles as a result of the drugs. After, say, 20 follicles are matured during a cycle, the attrition factor comes in to play. Out of 20 follicles, perhaps 15 of them will successfully yield eggs retrieved from the woman; out of those 15, maybe 11 of them will fertilize with the man's sperm in the culture dish; out of those 11, perhaps eight will have their cells divide correctly and they'll turn into viable embryos. Then the couple has eight possibly good embryos. They may decide to transfer three of them back into the woman, knowing that probably not all of them will implant to become clinical pregnancies; also, the more embryos put back, generally the greater chance of pregnancy. The five unused embryos (from the total of eight) can be frozen for a potential future attempt.

So if you are spending all of that money, time and effort, you want the most optimal results. For this, the fertility drugs are quite important. (Although, in some instances, IVF cycles are accomplished without the use of ovulation induction medications.) Also, since 1986, many clinics have suppressed women's menstrual cycles before the current IVF attempt month with contraceptive pills or an imitation hormone that disables the pituitary gland. The hormone suppression drug Lupron typically is used. And after the woman has her egg retrieval and embryo transfer, more drugs are needed: progesterone is prescribed to supplement the natural production of progesterone, aid in implantation and help with the early days of the embryo taking hold in the uterus. (Progesterone supplementation can be provided through injections, oral pills, a vaginal gel or vaginal suppositories, but the injections are considered the most effective.)

As a result of all this, going through IVF takes a lot of commitment. It may sound scary or overwhelming, but it's all manageable. It also helps to be educated about the whole process, so you know what you're getting into. But if you do the research, give it some serious thought and decide to make the IVF leap, your chances of having a successful MicroSort pregnancy are greatly increased.

Choosing a Clinic

Fortunately for couples who do not live near one of MicroSort's two current laboratories, it is not necessary to come to those locations to do IVF. Unlike with the IUI procedure, women don't have to find a hotel in Virginia and spend time away from home. You most likely won't have to leave your state for the IVF process, if you find a local physician (usually a reproductive endocrinologist) or fertility center that is a MicroSort collaborator or that may agree to become one.

Many MicroSort patients are now using these collaborating clinics in their own states for their IVF experience, although their husbands *are* encouraged to drive or fly out one time to Fairfax, Va. (or the new lab in Laguna Hills, Calif.), to make their contribution of a fresh semen sample for the sorting procedure. The sperm are then shipped to the local clinic after they've been processed and frozen by MicroSort. The local facility will thaw out the MicroSorted sperm when the sample is ready to be used in the IVF process.

If you use an outside fertility clinic for your MicroSort-IVF cycle, everything but the sperm sorting will be done at your local center. For a current list of MicroSort's IVF collaborators, see the organization's website or call its Collaborator Services number (both listed in appendix).

Adding ICSI

All MicroSort sperm that are sorted, frozen, shipped out of state and finally thawed for IVF must then go through a special step to achieve good pregnancy rates. Instead of leaving the sperm and eggs to find each other in the culture dish as in the standard IVF process, laboratory technicians working with MicroSorted sperm will do the process of intracytoplasmic sperm injection (ICSI), which increases fertilization success rates and is becoming more common in infertility clinics worldwide.

During ICSI, a single sperm is directly injected into an egg, leaving nothing to chance that egg and sperm will find each other. ICSI is typically done in standard IVF procedures when there is any male factor—when the prospective father's sperm count or motility is low or when there is some other sperm function or fertilization problem. ICSI is said to be one of the great infertility breakthroughs discovered in recent years (and it reportedly was discovered by accident!).

According to the experts at MicroSort, sperm that go through what MicroSort patients' sperm go through may need that extra boost—especially if they've been frozen and then thawed. ICSI costs an additional fee, but it also increases your chances of getting pregnant, so it may be well worth it. Most IVF-MicroSort patients have used ICSI to fertilize their eggs.

One collaborating clinic that uses ICSI to fertilize the eggs during an IVF-MicroSort cycle is the Cooper Center for In-Vitro Fertilization in Marlton, N.J., with Dr. Jerome H. Check as the collaborating physician. The center is well-known for its IVF program for infertility patients. "We perform well over 1,000 in-vitro egg retrievals per year and are one of the largest IVF programs in the United States," states the clinic.

I have met several women who have successfully gotten pregnant at the Cooper Center using the combination of IVF and ICSI with MicroSorted sperm. They were all seeking daughters and ended up getting them—some with twin girls.

A Story of Determination

New Jersey mother Yvette is one of those women. But first she went the easier route, as most MicroSort participants do—trying IUI at MicroSort.

"When I found out I was pregnant with my third son, I did some research on the Internet on gender selection," Yvette explains. "That is when I found their website and learned more about MicroSort. It sounded like the most reliable method out there (although I knew the pregnancy rate was low)."

Yvette and her husband began a roller-coaster ride of sorts. They drove down to Virginia three times to attempt IUIs with MicroSort. In her first attempt, Yvette took the oral fertility drug Clomid, but she only produced one follicle in time for her insemination, and no pregnancy resulted. "For the second and third attempts, I opted to try a more drastic approach and used injectibles to produce more follicles," she says. "I responded well to these. I used Gonal-F. I produced about seven or eight follicles each time. During my third IUI attempt, they could tell that at least one or two follicles had ruptured."

They thought their attempts were good ones, optimal for pregnancy—but the results were negative again. It was yet another blow, another hit on their savings account for nothing.

But not ready to give up their dream of a daughter, they started to think about the other method of conceiving with MicroSort: "I knew about IVF because two of my friends have used this method (not for gender selection). I had read about two women on the gender selection board who tried it along with MicroSort and were successful," Yvette explains. She had made lots of online friendships and learned about others' MicroSort experiences through iVillage's Parent Soup (see appendix).

"Since I didn't have any luck with the IUIs, I thought that this might be a more successful way to go since the egg would already be fertilized and I would just have to hope that implantation would take place. I also knew from using the injectibles that I would probably produce a fair amount of follicles." The same fertility drugs that are used in an injectible IUI cycle—such as Gonal-F—can be used for IVF.

"It was a tough decision, though, because it is costly and my medical insurance did not cover any of it except the meds," Yvette says. "I knew it would be my last attempt at gender selection since money was running out. I wanted my last attempt to be the best it could be."

Yvette and her husband were one of the first couples to consult with the Cooper IVF center to be a cooperating clinic with MicroSort. The center had already been doing some sex preselection of its own, and she says the Cooper staff were "very open to the idea of cooperating with MicroSort."

Yvette continues, "All of my questions were answered during my consultation and they even let me speak directly to the andrologist to find out more about the success of using frozen sperm. The doctors and nurses were very friendly and professional."

Fortunately, Yvette responded really well to the fertility protocol that the doctors put her on at Cooper. Things were looking up. On her retrieval day, the staff were able to extract a grand total of 39 eggs from her follicles. Her husband had driven earlier to Virginia to provide his sperm sample, and the sorted specimen was sent back home to New Jersey where it was thawed for fertilization of her eggs. Twenty of her retrieved eggs fertilized with the sperm through the ICSI procedure. The couple made the decision to have three of those resulting embryos put back into her uterus a few days after the retrieval. The rest were frozen, or cryopreserved.

Yvette's roller-coaster ride continued. After all that she had gone through, "I was unsuccessful for my first attempt." There was no pregnancy, only disappointment. However, "I was lucky enough to have frozen embryos left, so I did a frozen embryo transfer [FET] the following month." Because FETs have lower success rates, and the couple *really* wanted to conceive this time, they made the difficult decision to put four embryos back. They were prepared for the possibility of multiples, always a reality with IVF.

Two weeks later, Yvette had yet another pregnancy test. "That time, things worked out." She was pregnant! At the time, she was 35, and her sons were 6, 3 and 1. And there was just one baby inside her—a little girl, to be named Nicole.

Their roller-coaster ride was over. Nicole was born in 2002 to a huge family welcome. "My family feels complete now that our precious daughter is here. We felt blessed having our three wonderful sons, but had always wanted four children," says Yvette. "It was always a dream of mine to have a daughter. Finally, my dream has come true! Nicole is the sweetest little girl and brings us so much joy.

"I am so grateful to MicroSort for their technology and for helping us bring her into this world. All of the frustrations and heartache we faced during our gender selection journey was all worth it. We absolutely adore her ... including her big brothers. It's hard to believe Nicole is almost 2 years old. I still look at her every day and realize how lucky I am that she is my daughter. She is truly a miracle."

Costs at Cooper Center

The Cooper Center for IVF, where Yvette did both of her embryo transfers and where Nicole was conceived, is considered to be one of the more affordable IVF clinics in the United States. IVF is never cheap, but relatively speaking, Cooper's reasonable prices are one of the aspects that attract couples there for an IVF procedure. MicroSort participants find out about Cooper through the grapevine and its numbers for gender selection are increasing. (See appendix for the Cooper Center's contact information)

Here are Cooper's advertised prices (as of press time), and you can see if it's affordable:

- **Egg retrieval and embryo transfer, one cycle: $3,360**

(Or, natural-cycle IVF—no fertility medications pre-scribed: $1,800)
- **ICSI procedure—all eggs per one cycle: $775**

In addition to these charges, there are other expenses—some of which may be covered by your insurance company—for regular blood tests, pelvic ultrasounds and fertility medications (which are ordered separately). Costs will vary. And you will pay MicroSort separately for the sperm sorting (currently $2,300), for consultation ($100) and for sperm freezing, storage and shipping fees (which vary).

Other miscellaneous fees from Cooper:

- **New-patient comprehensive office visit: $230**
- **Frozen embryo transfer cycle (only necessary if first cycle fails): $1,600**
- **Cryopreservation of embryo(s) per cycle: $200**
- **Cryopreservation embryo maintenance for six months: $250**

IVF clinics in the United States reportedly all have a large number of cryopreserved embryos in storage. These can be saved for a couple's subsequent pregnancy attempt, they can be donated for embryo adoption or they may be discarded (a subject for ethical debate). There also has been a lot of heated public discussion about using these extra IVF embryos in medical research.

The Cooper clinic is just one of many MicroSort collaborators today. There are several more across the country, and some across the ocean. In Europe, some couples are sending sperm from local fertility clinics all the way to MicroSort in Virginia. The sperm are then sorted, frozen and shipped back to Europe where an IVF-ICSI procedure is carried out after the sperm are thawed. Although MicroSort states that the more optimal conditions involve working with fresh sperm, frozen sperm shipped from overseas for sorting remains an option. Several couples have successfully gotten pregnant in Europe in this manner, conceiving the babies they were seeking.

Costs at GIVF

Probably the *most* optimal option for the sperm in a MicroSort-IVF cycle is having everything done at Genetics & IVF Institute (GIVF) in Virginia, and some couples will travel to MicroSort's headquarters for this. There are a few advantages to this option, one being that the sperm never get frozen. The husband will provide his sperm right there in Fairfax, the sperm will immediately be processed and sorted by the MicroSort machine, and the sorted specimen will go directly to the adjacent IVF center for fertilization of the wife's eggs.

If a couple decide to use GIVF for both IVF and MicroSort, the price they pay will be a package deal, inclusive for IVF, ICSI and MicroSort. Following are the current prices (at press time) for such a combination cycle at GIVF, and some related expenses:

- **One IVF-ICSI fresh cycle using MicroSorted sperm: $12,200**
- **MicroSort patient consultation: $200**
- **Embryo freezing: $1,850**
- **Associated frozen embryo transfer cycle (only necessary if first cycle fails): $3,704**
- **Semen cryopreservation (per vial): $200**
- **Semen storage fees (per month): $34**

As with the prices at the Cooper Center, all medications are ordered and paid for separately (insurance companies may cover some of them). However, unlike Cooper's price list, GIVF's charge for an IVF-ICSI-MicroSort fresh cycle ($12,200) includes all ultrasounds and bloodwork as part of the regular cycle monitoring.

Costs at HRC

Another possibility, especially for couples who live on the West Coast, is to go to MicroSort's new location in California, a state that has had a high demand for gender selection. The Huntington Reproductive Center (HRC), a reproductive endocrinology and infertility practice with several locations in Southern California, has offered infertility services since 1988 and gender selection services (sperm spinning) since 1989. In October 2002, with public interest in sex selection rapidly growing, HRC took the big step of going into partnership with MicroSort; it now offers the new technology in its Laguna Hills center (Orange County, Calif.). The IVF clinic and MicroSort West are located in the same building, with a sorting machine on the premises—currently the only place in the world, other than MicroSort's headquarters in Virginia, with such technology.

Dr. Daniel A. Potter, a reproductive endocrinology specialist at HRC, is medical director for MicroSort West. "Many of us know someone who would desperately like to have a child of one gender or the other," he comments. "Perhaps a couple has one or more children of one gender already and would like to have another child—but would only consider doing so if the 50/50 odds could be shifted in favor of the other gender. Or, perhaps a couple already seeking fertility treatment has one child, and would prefer that the next child is the other gender if possible. Yet another couple may want to avoid passing a gender-linked genetic disease to their child.

"If a scientifically proven method of gender selection existed, most of these individuals would consider using it." Dr. Potter is there to help, by offering MicroSort services to such couples. He considers this technology the only "proven gender selection technology presently available."

For couples who would like to attempt IVF and MicroSort at the HRC location in Laguna Hills, here are the current costs (as of press time):

- **One regular IVF cycle: $5,900**
- **Low-cost program for two IVF cycles: $7,900 (if age 35 or under) or $8,400 (age 36–39)**
- **Low-cost program for three IVF cycles: $9,900 (if age35 or under) or $10,900 (age 36–39)**
- **MicroSort sperm sorting: $2,300**
- **ICSI procedure: $1,000**

Plus, patients will incur additional costs paying for such things as the initial consultation, the necessary medications and potential embryo freezing.

MicroSort patients at HRC also have the option of doing an IUI instead, although, like with the Virginia center, pregnancy rates are not as high. (For more information on HRC and MicroSort West, see the appendix for contact details.) Some MicroSort patients theorize that the success rate of three IUIs equals one IVF, and costwise, it often turns out to be about the same—so they may go directly to IVF, without spending time on the IUI. Others may not want to go through all that IVF entails. It's up to you.

MicroSort Overseas

MicroSort continues to expand and to add to its list of collaborators—fertility centers and physicians who work with

MicroSorted sperm in IVF-ICSI procedures in their home clinics.

"There are now more than 200 IVF program collaborators participating in the clinical trial around the world," says Dr. Keith Blauer, MicroSort clinical director. That number is expected to grow. To find out who is a collaborator and what parts of the country or world you may find one in, MicroSort's website will point you in the right direction (see the appendix).

One MicroSort collaborator can be found in London, where Dr. Peter Liu, an expert in sex selection, co-founded the London Gender Clinic in 1993. In 1997, he started collaboration with the Genetics & IVF Institute to help British couples with MicroSort sperm sorting, at the time a very new technology that was available. "As a result of this collaboration, we are proud to have assisted the first British couple to successfully preselect the sex of their baby (a healthy baby girl) in 1998 using the new MicroSort sperm separation technology," according to Dr. Liu.

He recently started collaboration with a number of IVF clinics outside the United Kingdom to make sex selection with IVF a reality for other families.

Dr. Liu comments that he is "happy for couples to consult him on the MicroSort sperm separation technology or in combination with IVF treatment for gender preselection." (See the appendix for his website.)

Another international collaborator is Professor Frank Comhaire of Ghent University Hospital in Belgium. He works with couples who come to him in Ghent to do gender preconception selection with IVF. He says that the husband provides the sperm at his clinic in Belgium, which Dr. Comhaire then has frozen and shipped to MicroSort in the United States, where it is sorted. "The sorted sperm is returned to Belgium and used for IVF." Dr. Comhaire does ICSI to fertilize the wife's retrieved eggs with the sorted sperm and then transfers the embryos back into her uterus. Patients have come to his clinic from several countries in Europe.

Dr. Comhaire is a proponent of preconception gender selection for family balancing (in which couples select the sex of their future child *before* conception). "The preconceptional method seems, to me, the best method for gender selection, since spermatozoa are not protected by law (they are not considered new or viable 'individuals' per se)," he comments. "In order to avoid sexism, the method is used exclusively for family balancing, more particularly to increase the probability of attaining a child of the 'missing' gender within the family."

Dr. Comhaire readily helps the European couples who come to him for this family balancing service. (See the appendix for his contact information.) For gender selection *after* conception, a more controversial practice, see chapter 9. Postconception selection (or gender determination) is carried out through the laboratory process of preimplantation genetic diagnosis (PGD).

Most MicroSort patients do *pre*conception sex selection, although a few may decide to find out the gender of their embryos after they are conceived, with PGD, and then specifically transfer back the embryos of the desired gender. My husband and I chose not to do PGD, instead counting on the MicroSort sperm sorting procedure to up our odds enough to get us our daughter. Read the next chapter for our IVF story.

CHAPTER

8

What It's Like To Go Through IVF

Our decision to go with IVF was not a quick or easy one. More than once in the past, I had said, "Oh, I wouldn't that," when I heard about the lengths some women went to get the baby they were looking for. I didn't think I could go through with IVF, with all that is involved. I was apprehensive about the process. Plus there was, of course, always the large amount of money to be risked. And, I was scared of the shots!

Well, a lot changed in a year and a half for me. I was not ever able to get pregnant with artificial insemination and MicroSort. Then, I developed secondary infertility problems related to fallopian tube blockage and an ectopic pregnancy, and even natural conception began to seem like an impossibility for me. My husband had more semen analysis tests done, and it looked like his fertility was declining, too. We considered adopting a little girl—for a while I did a lot of research on international adoption, focusing on South American countries. The information arrived that I sent out for, but the adoption process turned out to cost *more* money than a cycle of IVF; it would involve several weeks out of the country for my husband and me (difficult because of both job reasons and the logistics with our two boys); and, I still wanted a daughter of our own. I felt more comfortable knowing how she would start out in life, both in my womb and in early infancy; I wanted to breastfeed and I would like to know her genetic origins. But for those who adopt a child from another country,

I think it is a wonderful way to help someone less fortunate. And it could be the answer to a couple's dreams, as well.

For my husband and I, we found the answer to our daughter quest in our health insurance documents. One late night, after disparaging about our seeming infertility and the considerable difficulty of adoption, I lay in bed unable to sleep and depressed about giving up the dream of another baby. I suddenly had the idea of checking out our insurance coverage. In my home office that late night, I went to a desk drawer and pulled out the health insurance booklets, where I read that the company would cover 75 percent of IVF and ICSI plus a large percentage of the necessary medications. When I realized this fact—and the next day confirmed that my secondary infertility diagnosis would qualify us for coverage—I just knew that we had to give it a try. IVF is the perfect solution for a woman's tubal problems (which was one of the original purposes of this reproductive technology), and ICSI (discussed in chapter 7) is great for a lower sperm count. Plus, it was our solution to conceiving a daughter with MicroSort.

The answer seemed to fall right in my lap. And so I was off ....

For my IVF journey, I went right to the source. Living conveniently close to the Genetics & IVF Institute (GIVF) in Fairfax, my husband and I felt the best choice was to go with that center for our IVF, since GIVF is the developer of MicroSort. The company had a good reputation in our area, and I knew a few families who had successfully undergone IVF there—two for standard conception and one for gender selection. Their prices were considered pretty costly, but with our insurance coverage, we could afford one attempt with money from our savings. And the logistics of using MicroSorted sperm would be much easier at GIVF.

For me, going this route would possibly be my only way to conceive one last child, and especially a daughter. So I was willing to do whatever it took, whatever was involved. I read up to learn more about IVF, and although I had always had a slight fear of shots, I learned a lot of pain-relief tips from online friends who had undergone IVF and from infertility support boards on the Web. While before I had been a gender selection junkie, now I was an IVF fanatic. I learned everything that I could. And I decided that it was something that I could do.

Before beginning our IVF cycle, my husband and I sat down for a consultation with a reproductive endocrinologist at GIVF, where we went over our conception history, our previous MicroSort attempts and our desire to conceive a daughter, our particular fertility difficulties and what our plan would be for the upcoming cycle. The doctor recommended that we do ICSI, and we agreed. We also were invited to attend one of the free IVF classes held regularly at the institute.

My husband and I sat through the evening class with other couples and learned everything that was involved with an IVF cycle at GIVF. All of our questions were answered. The nurse-clinician leading the class discussed all the injections we would need to do, demonstrated how to do them and helped us all with a practice injection (husbands giving it to wives). We figured we were the only ones there doing MicroSort, and we didn't discuss that with anyone. We also were given a large binder to bring home that had step-by-step information to walk us through an entire cycle and included illustrated information sheets on what medications to take when, how to prepare and inject them, what was needed for the egg retrieval and what occurred during the embryo transfer, among other details.

IVF Protocols

There are two basic protocols for IVF patients at GIVF: "short-term Lupron" and "long-term Lupron." Lupron is a medication to prevent early ovulation that would interfere with the IVF cycle. For the long-term plan, patients start taking Lupron on day 21 of the month preceding their IVF cycle. Instead, I was assigned a short-term Lupron protocol, and I didn't have to start the drugs until the beginning of the current cycle.

On day 2 of my cycle (day 1 is the first day of the menstrual period), I arrived at GIVF's main offices, located in a building adjacent to MicroSort's headquarters. I checked in at the front desk, where I had to make payment for our cycle; I put our share of the cycle charge (including MicroSort) on our credit card, and we paid no additional fees other than the fertility drugs. The rest of the charges would be billed to our insurance company.

Then I went upstairs to the clinic rooms, where I underwent a "baseline" ultrasound to look at my ovaries and uterus, along with bloodwork to check my hormone levels. Everything looked normal, and I was good to go—and excited to start the journey!

That evening I began the Lupron injections—which are given with very small needles similar to the ones diabetics use for their regular shots (pretty painless). I had ordered all the medications in advance, from Freedom Drug, a low-cost mail-order pharmacy that had been recommended to me and can be accessed online or by phone. (I had consulted earlier with the GIVF staff on how much of the drugs to order.) Freedom Drug routinely deals with infertility patients and is very good with the details. They billed my insurance company for its share and put the remaining on my credit card; the shipping costs were free with a minimum purchase (easy to do with IVF cycles).

On the evening of day 3, we started the injections of follicle stimulating hormone (FSH). Those commonly used are Follistim, Repronex or Gonal-F; we went with Gonal-F, the "Cadillac of medications," according to the nurse-clinician we had consulted. So we figured this was the best. These shots were subcutaneous (into the skin rather than the muscle), so I wasn't too worried about them being painful. The best injection site for me was in my abdomen, where I would scrunch up a fatty fold of skin and my husband would quickly dart the needle in. For several days in a row, he gave me a Lupron shot in the morning and my FSH at night. (Many women learn how to do these shots themselves, but with my squeamish factor and my husband's skill with mixing and injecting the medication, it worked best if he did it.) After the first few injections it got easier, and we made it into our normal routine, at the same time every day. We even did the shots, furtively, in a friends' bathroom during a weekend gathering, in a car ride one night, and in a private restroom at an airport while traveling. Luckily nobody caught us! We didn't want to have to explain what we were doing.

During this time, my ovaries were being stimulated to grow multiple egg follicles, and I was monitored every couple of days by ultrasound to check their growth and with bloodwork to watch my hormone levels. We adjusted the FSH dosage as needed, according to the doctor's recommendations. I felt a little ill from the medications for a couple of days—like I had a type of flu—but that is normal, and it went away. Some women have no side effects from the drugs, according to an informal survey of my online IVF friends. However, some get uncomfortable, or bloated, as many follicles grow large on their ovaries; I never felt this problem. (There also is a rare but serious medical condition called ovarian hyperstimulation syndrome, or OHSS, which is excessive stimulation of the ovaries. IVF patients are warned about this potential problem, and what its symptoms are. If it does happen, the situation usually necessitates hospitalization. It typically worsens with pregnancy but can be treated, and it reportedly does not increase your chance of miscarriage. I knew of at least one woman whom this happened to. She was treated for it in the hospital and she and her baby ended up fine.)

As part of my regular monitoring, the nurse-clinicians also measured the thickness of my uterine lining during the ultrasound. A measurement over 10 is optimal; you want a nice fluffy lining that is thick enough for good implantation of the embryos when it comes time to place them in the uterus. My lining number never got to 10, it was always low—a fact that concerned me. I went on the IVF support boards and learned about some things I could do to try to increase my uterine-lining quality. (Eating fresh pineapple is rumored to be good for embryo implantation during IVF, so that is one thing I tried—it couldn't hurt!)

Eventually, after some days of going through my morning monitoring at GIVF, we noticed that my follicles were growing to the mature stage (anything measuring over 15 millimeters may contain mature eggs) and that my luteinizing hormone levels were indicating it was close to egg retrieval time. I did not have a whole lot of follicles, but my body was getting ready to ovulate, so we needed to get to the next step. I stopped the FSH injections (had already stopped the Lupron) and was instructed to have an hCG shot, to trigger the last step of egg maturation before the scheduled retrieval. The procedure was planned for a day and a half later.

The Retrieval

On our big day, I was not to eat or drink anything eight hours before the scheduled egg retrieval. That morning, my husband went to MicroSort to provide his semen contribution, which would undergo the sorting process in preparation for the retrieved eggs.

I was nervous about the retrieval; it is the most invasive part of the entire IVF cycle and the closest thing to surgery. GIVF has a lot of experience with transvaginal ultrasound-guided egg retrieval—having done it since 1985—but I didn't know what I would be experiencing.

That afternoon, I reported to the GIVF offices where I was given a comfortable room to wait in while I was prepared for my procedure. The doctor came in to answer any questions while I sat on a couch. I knew that they would soon put me in "conscious sedation," a sleeplike condition in which I was supposed to feel no pain. First I was given an injection of anti-nausea medicine and an IV for the other medications. From there I went to the retrieval room where I was helped onto the procedure bed and soon was "out."

During the egg retrieval—in which the physician delicately places a needle into each ovary and removes any mature eggs—I experienced dreaming under my sedation. I have to admit, in the "dream," I felt sharp sensations. I realized later it must have been the retrieval needle. I don't know if it was actual pain that I remember, but I definitely have memories of some sensation. However, most women I have talked to say that they were completely out for their retrieval and felt nothing at all. It probably depends on the woman as well as the clinic's methods and the amount, or type, of medication.

Although I did feel something under sedation during my retrieval, it was a procedure I would readily do again for the end result—and the worst was over! My husband drove me home and I took it easy for the rest of the day. I felt a little crampy that night, but it was nothing too bothersome. The next step was embryology, and I was excited about following the progress of any embryos that would be created by the ICSI process of my husband's sperm with my retrieved eggs. The embryology occurred in the GIVF lab for the next couple of days, and the staff keep the patients informed of the progress with daily phone calls. Unfortunately, only five eggs had been retrieved from my ovaries, but we hoped for every one of them.

The Transfer

My husband and I had already decided, in discussion with the doctor and with each other, that we would put back four

embryos (if possible). GIVF has its own stated recommendations, and it bases this on the woman's age and the number
and quality of embryos available. Here is GIVF's guidelines
for age and the number to transfer:

Age under 35—transfer *three* embryos
Age 35 to 39—transfer *four* embryos
Age 40 and up—transfer *four to eight* embryos

As we age, so do our eggs, and I knew that by 38 (my
age at the time), my eggs were not all of good quality. I had
already experienced two chemical pregnancies (very early
miscarriages) in the preceding year, and this was most likely
due to a chromosomal problem in each conception. I agreed
that out of four embryos transferred back to my uterus, there
would be a good chance of just one taking hold and becoming
a viable pregnancy. So four it would be.

After the ICSI process, four out of my five eggs had fertilized successfully—which I've been told was actually a good
ratio (the typical IVF fertilization rate is about 60 percent). If
we hadn't done ICSI, we might have had even fewer. So our
IVF cycle was very clear-cut: Put all of them back. We had no
embryos to freeze for later. All four of them were going to be
used that week in the transfer procedure. I was desperate that
it work—it was our only and last chance. The embryo transfer
was scheduled for two days after the retrieval. Most IVF
clinics schedule three-day transfers, but GIVF has found that
its success rates are just as good with a two-day transfer, so
that is what the staff usually does. (For another option, see the
adjacent box, "Blastocyst Transfer.")

Blastocyst Transfer

If several eggs (eight or more) are retrieved from a woman in an IVF cycle, a couple may have the option of doing a blastocyst transfer. This is a newer IVF technique in which the embryos are allowed to remain in the laboratory culture fluid for a total of five days, until their cell division advances to the blastocyst stage (with multiple cells). When this technique is used, the better embryos survive in the lab, and the weaker ones—or the ones with genetic defects—basically die off. Approximately half of the embryos that form on day 2 will die in culture by day 5, according to the Genetics & IVF Institute. The embryologists who are watching this process are then able to identify the high-quality embryos and select them for transfer. When those embryos are placed back in the woman's uterus, they typically have better implantation rates. With a regular IVF cycle—one in which the embryos are cultured in the lab for only two or three days before being replaced in the womb—there isn't a good way of knowing which of these embryos would survive and which wouldn't (a big part of the reason we transfer three or four at a time). Thus, the blastocyst process provides better success odds for each embryo than in a traditional transfer. As a result, fewer embryos need to placed back in the uterus after five days, because the chances of each one developing into a baby are higher.

When a couple decides to go forward with a day 5 blastocyst transfer—and this is something that is being done at GIVF, among other clinics—the standard recommendation is to put back only two embryos, regardless of maternal age. Because the blastocysts have a higher implantation rate, fewer embryos are needed to achieve pregnancy, and the great benefit? Fewer multiple births. Couples who put back three, four or more embryos run the risk of triplets, quadruplets or higher—a low risk, but a risk nonetheless. And the higher order of multiples, the more dangerous the pregnancy—for the mother and, especially, for the babies. When you put back two embryos, you only run the risk of conceiving twins (for some parents a welcome idea). So more couples are going for the blastocyst transfer, if it is possible in their circumstances—and some clinics are recommending this process.

In my case, I did not have enough embryos to go through with a blastocyst transfer, since I only had four to work with. Despite the benefits of a day 5 blastocyst transfer, it is riskier when you're only dealing with a few embryos; you are putting all of your hopes on just a handful. Some of the embryos that die in the lab culture between days 2 and 5 may actually have implanted if they were transferred at an earlier stage, into the natural environment of the uterus. And with my advanced age, there was more of a risk in leaving the embryos in the lab for so many days. Since I would have none to freeze from this cycle, I wanted to get them all transferred earlier. If they failed to divide properly in the lab culture over those five days, I would be left with nothing to transfer back. My doctor agreed that blastocyst transfer probably would not be the best decision in our circumstances. But for younger women who perhaps produce a lot of eggs, this technique may be very beneficial. I have known couples who underwent this procedure successfully, and it is probably something worth looking into—especially if you're worried about multiples.

My embryo transfer was scheduled for Halloween 2001—both a trick and a treat. It meant that I wouldn't be able to take my two little boys trick-or-treating (who at this point were 2½ and just-turned-5). My husband would bring them out, while I was expected to take it easy on the family room couch. And if a pregnancy took, I would always know that I had a Halloween conception, a fun hallmark to mark the exact day that my future daughter took hold inside me. So I was ready for a different kind of Halloween.

That day, while kids all around town were getting into their costumes and getting ready for fun, I drove myself to the GIVF building for my embryo transfer. Our four embryos had continued dividing in the lab (the more cells they reach, the better), and we had been given their embryo quality scores (or grades), which showed two of them of better quality than the other two. We were putting all four of them back. If we had had several to pick from, we would have chosen the four best-quality ones, which is the common procedure at GIVF. However, I was told that the quality scores do not predict birth defects. We just hoped that out of the four, one would be perfect and turn into our little girl.

I arrived in the clinical waiting room with a full bladder, as instructed. This was the only requirement for the transfer day. I had consumed several glasses of water before the drive over there. So a little uncomfortable, I walked into the procedure room for the big event.

I climbed up onto the procedure bed and got into the typical pelvic exam position, as directed. I knew that the procedure would feel similar to the artificial inseminations I had undergone previously, and they were not painful. Both processes are similar to a pelvic exam, and although I would be totally awake for this IVF procedure, I was not apprehensive. (I *was* eager to empty that bladder soon, though!)

My doctor and a nurse-clinician were both there, and they explained everything that would be happening. A speculum was inserted and I was prepared for the transfer. The usual ultrasound screen was nearby for viewing everything. In the back wall in front of me, a sliding half-door opened and an embryologist was behind it, in the embryology lab. (Surprise! I didn't even know that was there.) She had loaded our four little embryos into a catheter and then formally announced the number and identity of the embryos as she carefully passed the catheter over to the doctor. I felt a little exposed because everybody was down in front of my open legs—but what can you do! This is the way IVF works. After all my monitoring and procedures over the past weeks, I knew I couldn't be too concerned anymore about modesty. I just wanted to get pregnant.

Under the guidance of the ultrasound equipment, the doctor gently slid the catheter of embryos up and into the top of my endometrial cavity (at the uterus), and the tiny little embryos were ejected from the catheter. Everything played out on the ultrasound screen. The doctor removed the catheter and handed it to the embryologist, who checked to make sure that all the embryos were out of it. They were.

I was instructed to lay on the procedure bed, with my legs slightly raised, for 30 minutes. The staff made sure I was comfortable. I had been told earlier that I could have a urinary catheter (to empty my bladder) after the transfer if I was really uncomfortable, but I decided that I could wait to use the bathroom if I didn't move at all. I just laid there and willed those embryos to start burrowing in!

My husband and sons had arrived and were waiting for me in the clinic's waiting room. Rather than trying to get a baby-sitter for the boys in the middle of the day (and to have to try to explain why), we had decided that he would stay home with them until it was time to pick me up. After my 30 minutes post-transfer were up, I ran to the bathroom (ah, relief!) and then out to the waiting room. My husband drove us home and I tried to take it easy the rest of the day, to stay horizontal as much as possible to let those embryos take hold. (The hardest part was what to do about trick-or-treaters at our door when my family was out collecting their own treats!)

That week I started the required progesterone shots, which were intramuscular (in the muscle) instead of subcutaneous. This was the part that I had been dreading the most. They had to go into the hip/buttock area, every night, and the needle was bigger than the subcutaneous ones that we had used for the FSH injections. But I had my computer printout list of pain relief tips I had collected, and I obsessively tried every one. For example, we would initially warm the thick progesterone-in-oil substance with a heating pad (to make it go in easier) and cool the injection site with an ice pack to make the area numb before injection. After my husband injected the medication, I put the heating pad on the spot where it had gone in, and that seemed to help a little. I did end up with some bruising, however (as I did with the FSH shots, too)—but that is all par for the course, and it eventually goes away.

We soon found out from the MicroSort lab that our sorting procedure had yielded a sperm sample of 95.6 percent "X" purity—our best MicroSort purity ever! This meant that almost 96 percent of the sperm collected and available for ICSI was female producing. We had a very good chance that all four of the embryos placed back in me were girls. Now we just needed to find out if at least one took and I was pregnant.

The Verdict

We were instructed to wait 14 days after the retrieval to do a pregnancy test. It was hard for me to wait that long—I could hardly think about anything else—and so of course I started earlier. I had been warned that the hCG shot that I had taken could still be in my system and may provide a false positive on a home pregnancy test (HPT) before the 14 days were up. My plan was to start doing HPTs at 11 days after retrieval (which is comparable to ovulation); some tests on the market now claim to start working that soon after ovulation. I figured that if I was pregnant, the HPTs would slowly get darker; if it was just the hCG shot that the test was picking up, that line would slowly fade with time each day. I hoped that this was a good plan.

I got a positive HPT at the 11-day mark. I was cautiously excited. Each morning, I did another test (always the same brand), and the HPTs showed lines that consistently got darker each day. My excitement was growing; I wanted this *so* much.

Every morning I called my husband at work with the latest on my HPT obsession.

On day 14, I reported to GIVF for a scheduled blood pregnancy test in the morning. That afternoon, they called with the results: I was definitely pregnant, I had a beta hCG level of 156. That was a nice high number. I couldn't believe it! I was so excited. When I had had my chemical pregnancies in the past, my numbers were much lower. This was a good sign. The higher the number, apparently, the less of a chance of miscarriage. I was told to come back in three days, to see if my levels had more than doubled, which was an indication of a healthy pregnancy.

At 17 days past retrieval, my beta hCG level was 948! Very high. Not only had it doubled, but it had increased by six times in those three days. I was ecstatic. But, of course, with a number that high, I had to start worrying about multiples, always a possibility with an IVF transfer of four embryos. They told me to make an appointment for an ultrasound in two weeks—then we would find out what I had in there.

Two weeks later, I drove back to GIVF, tired and slightly queasy—both good signs, as the receptionist commented. I went to the examining room, excited but nervous. The nurse-clinician found two yolk sacs in my uterus on the ultrasound screen—the beginnings of two possible babies. However, one of them ("sac B") looked empty. It was hard to tell this early. The doctor said I should return one week later to confirm. Would I have twins, or a singleton?

My next ultrasound showed only one yolk sac, and it was measuring just right for where I should be in the pregnancy (7 weeks gestation). The doctor said that the other embryo probably just "fizzled out," or what is known as vanishing twin syndrome. This is common in IVF pregnancies, and it really did not upset me. I had barely even gotten used to the idea of twins, and I knew from the first ultrasound that it was unlikely that sac B was a viable pregnancy. When I got home, I did some Internet research on this occurrence, and I learned that sometimes the body just absorbs the vanishing twin, and other times it bleeds it out. So I was prepared for any bleeding, as scary as that might be.

But what this whole thing had taught me was that our decision to put back four embryos was the right one for us. Out of the four, two did not implant at all, one fizzled out and one remained, to grow and become a baby. If we had only put back three embryos, I may not have been pregnant. After all of that money, the time, the shots, the procedures, the emotion invested, everything—I really wanted to optimize our chances of a successful pregnancy. I was so glad we put back four. Some people had thought that might be too many—and we did realize our risk of multiples—but for me, especially at my age, it was just the right number. That choice may have been what made our IVF venture successful—and, finally, we had good luck with MicroSort.

The Baby

My pregnancy continued pretty uneventfully—a huge relief to me. I did have a couple instances of very light bleeding, or "spotting," and when that happened I hoped it was the vanishing twin and not a complication for the baby. Everything seemed fine with the pregnancy, so we were optimistic that we would have a daughter. I continued the progesterone shots until I was 10 weeks pregnant—at that point, the placenta was formed and producing what was needed and it was safe to discontinue the shots. That was a big relief—I was so happy to stop the shots forever. It took a few weeks for the bruises on my buttocks to fade and go away, and for me to be able to jog without pain at the bruised sites. But, again, it was all worth it for the chance to finally make my dream come true.

After my second ultrasound at GIVF, I had "graduated" from the clinic and was released to my regular obstetrician for medical care. He knew that the pregnancy was the result of IVF but I didn't tell him about MicroSort; it really wasn't necessary information for the care of the pregnancy. At 20 weeks gestation, my OB sent me for the routine ultrasound that almost all pregnancies nowadays have. I was excited to finally find out if the baby I was carrying was indeed a girl. I knew there was about a 5 percent chance that it was a boy, and I had to be prepared for that possibility. (I had a favorite boy name just in case!)

Wouldn't you know it, this baby would not cooperate. After years of researching gender selection, and months of trying different methods, of many attempts at pregnancy and everything I'd been through with IVF—I finally was at the point of finding out, and my baby was being modest. We could not see between the legs, as much as the ultrasound physician tried to get a good view and I tried to jiggle the baby around. I was getting frustrated!

The doctor suggested I go into the waiting room while he saw another patient, and maybe the baby would eventually change positions. We knew the baby was healthy—everything had checked out—and that was a relief. But I just couldn't leave without knowing whether I had a "he" or a "she" in there. So I agreed to wait and come back in later. The doctor did not know this was a MicroSort baby, but luckily he was patient with me and had agreed to give it another try.

Later on, I hopped back on the ultrasound table, and we gave it another go. This time, the doctor saw it, the three white lines indicating female genitalia. "It looks like a girl," he said: the words I had been waiting forever to hear. He couldn't be 100 percent sure—they never are with ultrasounds—but I took home those words and played them over and over. It had finally happened. My husband and I had conceived a daughter, most likely, and soon she would be with us. I could go out and buy pink.

In July 2002, Rachel Natalie was born. She was, indeed, all girl. I couldn't believe it—changing her diaper, there was no little penis there, ready to squirt up at me. I had to get used to changing a girl's diapers. It was amazing, and unreal, and something I had at one point almost give up on as ever happening for me. And although I love my sons more than anything in the world, I am so happy to have a daughter. I love dressing her up in little dresses and bows. I am glad to no longer be the only female in the family. I love seeing her with her brothers and father, who adore her. I am glad I will have this little girl to raise into a woman. There is something now complete for me, the missing puzzle piece has been put into place.

My long-dreamed-of picture of a little girl posing between her brothers has become a reality. This could happen for you, too, if you would like to try the same journey. MicroSort in combination with our first stab at IVF did it for us.

Now there is also a new technique that basically will guarantee gender, if you do get pregnant. To learn about this method, and another woman's success story, see the next chapter.

CHAPTER

9

Adding PGD to the Mix

What is the only sure way of predetermining the gender of your baby? There is a way to do it, and this chapter tells you how. Over the past few years, a new method of sex selection has emerged that brings couples the closest thing to a 100 percent guarantee for choosing the gender of their offspring.

With the turn of the new century came a new idea for gender selection: preimplantation genetic diagnosis (PGD). Although this technology was available at some fertility clinics in the 1990s, PGD was only done for medical reasons, such as avoiding cystic fibrosis. Increasingly, more clinics around the world are beginning to do it, or at least consider it, for the purposes of gender selection (basically, "family balancing"). In the past few years, PGD has stepped into the spotlight for gender determination, but not without controversy.

PGD essentially is embryo selection. It can be used as a postconception type of gender selection. After the egg and sperm are united and create an early embryo, that embyro can be biopsied for chromosomal or genetic disorders before being placed back in the womb. It also can be tested for gender. If a couple decides to have an IVF cycle and only put back the embryos of a particular gender, they are choosing some and "rejecting" others due to gender. This has more ethical considerations than preconception selection methods such as MicroSort, in which the sperm are sorted out and selected *before* the conception of an embryo.

To make it a little more complicated—or, to give couples yet another option—PGD can be done in combination with MicroSort. This is an additional (and more costly) choice that MicroSort patients may select if they go to an IVF clinic that will perform PGD for such purposes. In this way, couples can opt to find out the gender of their embryos before they are implanted in the womb. (This can only be done with IVF, not IUI.) PGD reportedly will give MicroSort patients that 100 percent guarantee that the embryos they create in the lab and select for implantation are all female (or, conversely, all male) when transferred into the uterus. MicroSort by itself, although it can produce 90 percent success rates for baby girls, is not as foolproof as PGD; you could still end up with a boy. You know what you're getting if you do PGD. But without MicroSort, it is more difficult to produce enough embryos of the desired gender, so PGD may not always work (or, get to the point of embryo transfer and pregnancy). Confused yet?

Let's look at it this way: Couples who are interested in doing IVF for gender purposes basically have three choices—(1) MicroSort alone, (2) PGD alone, or (3) MicroSort plus PGD. For couples seeking a daughter, the first choice will give them a majority of female embryos (if the woman responds well to the IVF protocol). The second choice may produce a significantly smaller proportion of female embryos, but they will know for sure that they are selecting those embryos for transfer into the uterus.

The third choice, however, gives the couples the best odds of success. This combination of technologies will cost the couple the most money, but they can be confident that MicroSort will produce a high ratio of female embryos (like nine out of 10), and they will know that PGD guarantees that those female embryos will be the ones selected for uterine implantation. And for couples looking for a boy, the same applies, although they may not have 90 percent male embryos to choose from, more likely closer to 75 percent. Thus, MicroSort and PGD together are the most effective method of selecting a baby's gender.

Genetics & IVF Institute (GIVF), the parent clinic of MicroSort in Fairfax, Va., offers PGD in combination with MicroSort. So does the Huntington Reproductive Center in Southern California, which also has the MicroSort technology on-site. Some other infertility clinics are starting to offer PGD for couples undergoing IVF for family balancing—with or without MicroSort sperm. The Fertility Institutes, with centers in Los Angeles, Las Vegas and Mexico, will do IVF with MicroSort or PGD; they advertise for clients on the Web (see appendix for their contact information). And from as far away as India, the Malpani Infertility Clinic in Bombay will perform PGD for parents who want to find out gender (also in the appendix).

The PGD Process

How is PGD done? Well, once the eggs are retrieved from the woman and fertilized with sperm in the laboratory, the resulting embryos are cultured and they start to cleave, or divide, in a petri dish. After they reach the eight-cell stage, typically the third day in the IVF process, they are ready for biopsy. The technician is able to tease off one of their cells (blastomeres) for molecular diagnosis. He or she does this by holding the embryo in position with a holding pipette, under microscopic observation, and using a glass needle to drill a hole through the outer layer. The technician then removes a single cell by gentle suction. This process takes a highly skilled, precise ability and involves the coordination and dedicated experience of several staff members. Not all IVF clinics are qualified to do PGD. There are a limited number of centers with PGD services in the world (approximately 50 at press time), although that number appears to be growing.

During the subsequent analysis of the embryo's cell, some significant genetic abnormalities can be identified, in which case that particular embryo would be ruled out for possible transfer into the uterus. Those early embryos that appear to have normal chromosomes will be available for implantation or they can be cryopreserved (frozen) for future use. While the single blastomeres are being tested, the embryos are kept in culture and allowed to further divide; they usually have to be cultured to the blastocyst stage (see chapter 8 for details) and transferred around day 5.

For gender purposes, an embryo's cell also can be tested for the presence or absence of a Y chromosome. Thus the technician discovers, before the embryos are selected for implantation, which are male and which are female.

PGD was not created for balancing the gender of families, but rather for preventing medical problems, such as X-linked diseases. The technology was a great breakthrough for physicians to be able to identify genetic diseases in embryos before attempting a pregnancy from IVF. "PGD was developed for patients who were at risk of having children with serious genetic disorders, such as hemophilia, which often discouraged them from having their own biological children. These couples are often faced with attempting a type of 'Russian Roulette' to have children, many times having to confront the difficult decision to terminate an affected pregnancy," according to Healthlibrary.com.

"Consider a woman known to be carrying the gene for hemophilia. She has a 50 percent risk of an affected male in each pregnancy. While her daughters have a 50 percent risk of being carriers, they are going to be clinically normal. She may not wish to become pregnant if she has to make decisions about an affected child in a viable pregnancy. However, she would become pregnant if she knew she had conceived a daughter—and with PGD, this possibility becomes a reality.

PGD thus eliminates the need for possible pregnancy termination after prenatal diagnosis of a fetus with hemophilia."

As a result, PGD is an important tool for battling sex-linked diseases. (See adjacent box, "PGD's Contributions.") A woman who carries a gene for a particular disease can guarantee that her future child will not be of the gender that may be afflicted with the disorder. And there are more of these disorders than most people know. "Some 370 genetic abnormalities are known to be X-linked, recessive disorders that are generally expressed by male children born to women possessing an X-chromosome with the defective gene," according to a "Human Sex Preselection" article in *The Journal of New Developments in Clinical Medicine* (1998, Vol. 16, No. 2). "Since most female children do not exhibit the X-linked recessive disorder, it would be advantageous for a woman known to be a carrier of such an X-linked recessive gene to employ female sex preselection to avoid the birth of a son who would express the genetic condition."

As the story of such a disorder is related in chapter 5, the birth of such a child could be heartbreaking for all involved, and gender selection is the modern-day solution. PGD appears to be the best method for that solution.

With the benefit of PGD, couples can choose their embryos for both health purposes and for the desired sex. More clinics are starting to perform PGD for family balancing in the United States (and probably internationally), although they may not publicize this fact. In a few cases that I have learned about, the couple consulted a local IVF clinic that is known to do PGD for medical purposes (e.g., for families that carry genetic diseases or for older women with an increased chance for chromosomal disorders) and asked if the staff would consider doing it for gender purposes. One woman in New England, who was in her upper 30s, mentioned her age as a reason to check for chromosomal problems but also asked if the clinic would do the PGD test for gender as well and select the female embryos for transfer. The clinic agreed, but only if the female embryos were of equal or better quality than the male embryos. For good reason, fertility clinics' number-one priority is to transfer healthy embryos back into the woman, so that there is a lesser chance of miscarriage and a greater chance of a healthy baby (and this gives them better IVF success rates).

But if a couple's IVF cycle has produced three good male embryos and three good female embryos—all seeming of equal quality—why not select the three of the less represented gender in the family to put back? That is what some couples are asking for.

PGD's Contributions

This book is mainly about gender selection for family balancing, but the origin of the PGD method is related to technology advances in the prevention of genetic disorders and disease. The Huntington Reproductive Center (HRC) in Southern California has been on the forefront of these and other human reproduction technologies. HRC, which is committed to providing PGD technology to couples at risk of having a genetically abnormal baby, offers PGD for both medical and gender purposes. (See the appendix for HRC's contact information.) This West Coast IVF center has been following the latest research on PGD.

"In recent years, significant advances in technology have enabled researchers to trace many disorders and diseases to their roots in the genetic code. Chromosome stretches, or even isolated genes, can now be used as markers to identify individuals at risk for certain illnesses," according to Dr. Barry Behr and Victor Ivahnenko on the HRC website.

"A normal embryo has 22 pairs of chromosomes called autosomes and one pair of sex chromosomes (XX or XY)," they explain. "Embryos that do not carry the normal pair of each chromosome are called aneuploids. Those that contain three copies of a particular chromosome (trisomy) are the cause of some genetic disorders such as Down's syndrome (trisomy 21).

"Abnormal aneuploid embryos, either with monosomy (one missing) or trisomy (an extra one), are usually normal in appearance. It is not possible to distinguish these morphologically from other embryos. It is only through genetic analysis that they can be differentiated. Without such an analysis, many of these embryos are unknowingly transferred to patients. Depending on the specific abnormality, in IVF pregnancies, research has shown that chromosomal abnormalities such as aneuploidies of the embryo increase either the risk of spontaneous miscarriage, the development of a genetically abnormal child or no pregnancy at all."

Thus, PGD provides a great benefit in identifying those abnormal embryos and helping reproduction professionals select the embryos with the greatest chance of turning into a healthy child. Women with a history of recurrent miscarriages may especially benefit: "Selective implantation of embryos with normal chromosome compliments have also been shown to result in high pregnancy rates with decreased spontaneous miscarriage rates," according to HRC.

And for women who are carriers of certain genetic disorders, PGD is invaluable. "PGD was first employed in 1989 with subsequent birth of normal females to couples at risk of various X-linked recessive diseases. The number of genetic diseases potentially diagnosable by PGD is vast." HRC lists examples of such disorders: chromosomal translocations, Turner syndrome, DiGeorge syndrome, cystic fibrosis, Fancony anemia, fragile X syndrome, hemophilia A, Huntington disease, sickle cell anemia, Tay-Sachs disease and many more.

Safety of PGD

As with any new medical technology, there is always the question of safety. Some couples may be concerned that removing a single blastomere from an early embryo and then transferring that embryo into the potential mother could result in the future baby having an abnormality. However, it is reported that neither the risk of miscarriage nor the risk of birth defects is increased with PGD. At such an early stage of the embryo, each cell is "totipotential," and it is able to give rise to a complete embryo by itself.

"The genetic material of the embryos (which is derived from both parents) is not altered in any way during a PGD cycle, and early embryological development is similar to natural conception, except that it occurs in the laboratory," according to Dr. Harvey J. Stern in the *Genetics & IVF Institute Newsletter* (Fall 2001). "At this early stage of embryological development, the blastomeres have not yet become committed to form cells of a specific organ or tissue and are capable of becoming any type of cell. Removal of a small number of cells of the early embryo does not decrease the ability of that embryo to become a complete, normal fetus and child.

"Data from many years of PGD in animals and over 500 lives births in humans indicates that PGD does not lead to an increase in birth defects or chromosomal disorders."

The Genetics & IVF Institute is currently (as of press time) offering IVF patients a deal in which, if the couple qualify for the MicroSort clinical trial and desire PGD, the cost of the MicroSort sperm separation will be free. So they pay extra for PGD but not for MicroSort. The current charge at GIVF's Virginia headquarters is $16,200 for the whole package—including IVF, ICSI (explained in chapter 7), PGD and MicroSort. Patients pay that same price whether they participate in the MicroSort clinical trial or whether they do the PGD without MicroSort (not all couples qualify for MicroSort). Regardless of which way you go, the cost of medications is additional.

One Family's Experience

Margaret of Massachusetts is one woman who went for the complete package to bring home a daughter. Like many couples who end up trying high-tech gender selection, she and her husband had initially attempted the Shettles method of timing intercourse to conceive a girl. She had worked diligently over the years to figure out her ovulation time with ovulation predictor kits and to concentrate on changing her internal environment. The result was always a boy. She had three of them.

"I was convinced it worked, which made the news of 'It's a boy' that much more devastating," says Margaret of her third pregnancy. As much as she loved her boys, she couldn't give up the hope for a daughter.

Then she learned about MicroSort, when her sister showed her information she had gotten from the Internet. "I couldn't believe it was only offered in Virginia at first, and I wondered how I could pull it off going all that way," Margaret relates. From her home in Massachusetts, the drive to MicroSort's office in Fairfax, Va., is about eight hours long.

But she was intent on conceiving a girl, so she and her husband made the effort to go to Virginia to attempt MicroSort with artificial insemination (or IUI). Margaret daily took 100 mg of the oral fertility drug Clomid, as directed. She made two complete IUI attempts—both ended up negative, no pregnancy. On her third attempted cycle, she developed a "huge" cyst on one of her ovaries (which occasionally occurs due to the Clomid) and had to cancel the cycle before the IUI.

As a result, Margaret had to take a break from trying to conceive and get rid of the cyst. "This made me take several months off from MicroSort," she explains. "During these months, I began to learn how really low the pregnancy rate was with IUI. I knew that if I could gain my husband's support, IVF was the way to go." She had done her research and knew that IVF attempts had a significantly higher pregnancy rate than doing IUI (some data show IVF success rates per cycle at about 35 percent, while MicroSort IUIs are much lower, closer to 18 percent). "So I put the money from the third cycle toward my IVF attempt."

During Margaret's research, she had learned about PGD. "Once we made the decision to go the IVF route and we knew GIVF would do PGD just for gender selection, we figured— why not? My husband remembers how devastated I was to hear boy number 3 and wasn't willing to take that 10 percent chance of boy. We knew we were taking a chance at having twins when doing IVF, so with PGD we knew at least that they'd be girls."

Thus Margaret and her husband made the big decision to do IVF with MicroSort and PGD at GIVF. It was a serious commitment, because of the time involved in an entire IVF-PGD cycle and the location of GIVF eight hours away from their home—not to mention the money they'd have to lay out. But they wanted to give their attempt the best possible odds of success, and they figured doing it all at GIVF in Virginia would be the answer.

In February 2002, when Margaret was 34 and her boys were 6½, 4½ and 1½, she took time off from her part-time job and loaded the whole family into the car to drive down to Virginia. The prospective father contributed his sperm sample. Margaret had already been on the FSH protocol to stimulate her ovaries for IVF and she was getting ready for the egg retrieval. After it, her husband and kids would go back home to Massachusetts. Alone in the hotel in an unfamiliar town away from everybody, her cell phone was her connection for keeping in touch with family and friends and to follow directions from GIVF. But, fortunately, things were going very well with her IVF cycle.

As needed for PGD and a day 4 embryo transfer, the staff at GIVF were able to obtain several eggs from Margaret's ovaries—they retrieved 15 eggs, and fertilized 11 of them. Through phone calls with the GIVF lab and with her husband, she made the decision to put back three of the embryos, two of which had made it to the morula stage (an advanced stage one step before blastocyst) by day 4.

Their MicroSort purity rate for X-bearing sperm was 90.5 percent, just as one would expect. The even better news? All 11 of the embryos were girls, according to the PGD results. So Margaret knew that the three embryos being transferred to her uterus were all female. If she were to get pregnant, all the money was worth it—she and her husband had the 100 percent girl guarantee they had wanted.

After her embryo transfer, Margaret returned by train to her home, trying to take it easy and give her brand-new embryos a chance to stick. It worked. Two weeks later she found out she was pregnant, and soon after that she and her husband discovered they were going to have twins. Twin girls. In November 2002, the girls were born, and life has not been the same.

"All I can say is that my life is now complete," Margaret concludes. "I always felt that something was missing. There is nothing quite like having a 'balanced' family. It has made my husband a more sensitive man and to view all things in life more differently now that he has daughters.

"I, myself, feel not so *alone* in a house of males. I used to get easily irritated by the rambunctious behavior and sports-oriented life of boys, but now I enjoy boys being boys. I cherish every moment with my girls. I don't think I will ever take them for granted. I hope to someday have the special mother-daughter bond that I have with my mom."

Margaret's words could be my own, so close they are to my own feelings and emotions. And many more women feel this way, too. If you do, PGD is a possible option for your gender search. Of course, financing is always an issue, and IVF-PGD is not inexpensive. Some families feel that it is worth it, though—to borrow from their savings, use up credit cards or take out loans for the sake of a dream. When compared to the costs of adoption—or of continually conceiving (and then raising) more children in the hopes of getting that missing gender—high-tech gender selection may seem like a viable option. Margaret and her husband certainly thought so.

Facts About PGD

Even though PGD can help eliminate some diseases in future offspring and is a method for providing couples with a gender guarantee, there still is no guarantee of pregnancy with a laboratory attempt using IVF and PGD. All IVF technology, however efficient it is at producing embryos in vitro in the lab, still cannot make a baby take hold in the uterus. After the embryos are transferred back to the womb, even if they have been tested with PGD (and not all PGD gender tests also test for health—this is an extra step), there still is a chance for no pregnancy, or of miscarriage. All couples going into a cycle of IVF and PGD need to realize this. Sometimes the fate of an IVF cycle is all up to chance—no matter how fortuitous the cycle seems to be and how good the embryos appear. This book has detailed some IVF success stories, but there also are IVF failures, some unexplainable.

However, the technology is always improving, the techniques are always evolving and most likely the implantation rates of embryos that go through IVF and PGD will improve in the near future. There are a couple of important factors for a successful IVF-PGD cycle. The first is to produce a lot of follicles during the ovarian stimulation phase—so that there are several eggs to fertilize, many embryos to biopsy, and enough good blastocysts to choose from for embryo transfer. Retrieving at least 10 eggs is optimal—especially if a couple is aiming for a certain gender without doing MicroSort, so that they can be assured of at least two or three healthy embryos of the desired sex.

An important factor for attaining a healthy pregnancy is being able to rule out chromosomal problems in the embryos. Approximately 60 percent of all naturally occurring reproductive losses in pregnancies are estimated to be caused by chromosomal abnormalities. Women of advanced maternal age undoubtedly have a higher incidence of chromosomal abnormalities in their eggs. With PGD testing, the embryos that are produced with their partner's sperm can be screened for certain anomalies and only the ones that appear normal selected for implantation. The more eggs that can be retrieved in their IVF cycle, the better chance of finding some good, healthy embryos. PGD also may benefit women with infertility problems and/or recurrent miscarriages. Having a physician closely monitor the patient is paramount, so that the IVF protocol is able to produce the maximum number of eggs for the most successful cycle without causing ovarian hyperstimulation syndrome (explained in chapter 8).

Another fact to consider is that there are always biological variables inherent in the PGD process. Not every IVF cycle will produce embryos that can be perfectly biopsied. Some cells may not give a clear "signal" when being analyzed, or it may not be possible for the technician to interpret the signals clearly. I heard from one woman, who was close to 40 when attempting IVF-PGD, who said that the PGD testing did not work on the embryos in one of her cycles. Her embryologists were not able to extract information from the blastomeres; in essence, they could not get communication from the cells.

She ended up canceling that cycle and attempting another one a few months later, which fortunately *was* successful and she ended up getting pregnant.

Again, these types of problems may become surmountable in the future as the technology improves. Over the years, I have continued to learn about yet another new, amazing technology or about more couples' experiences with overcoming obstacles and getting pregnant or achieving the gender they were seeking. The stories of fertility breakthroughs and new frontiers in technology throughout the past couple of decades have been nothing short of phenomenal.

As the technology becomes even more advanced and the word gets out about PGD, the rate of people trying this process should only go up. In a little more than a decade, the number of couples trying PGD for medical purposes—and for success stories to occur—already has increased. And the use of PGD for family balancing will probably become more common as more clinics in more parts of the world join in.

The acceptance of PGD for pure gender reasons, however, is not in the mainstream yet—nor may it ever be. In Europe, PGD for gender purposes is illegal in some countries. In other countries, however, couples have had it done to conceive the child of their choice. Some people have traveled from one European country to another to have IVF-PGD performed for family balancing (without MicroSort). I have heard from at least three women who did this, and they succeeded, if not on the first try then on subsequent ones. (Understandably, these women keep their identities secret and the details of their IVF-PGD providers low-key.) The cost of assisted reproduction technology to patients in Europe appears to be lower than it is in the United States, and some couples will do IVF-PGD more than once until sufficient numbers of embryos of the desired gender are produced and selected for clinical transfer. Those not selected can be cryopreserved. However, this type of PGD use is still very controversial.

PGD is a great technology for couples with inherited X-linked disorders and for women with increased risks of miscarriage—but it will continue to be debated, both in the United States and worldwide, about its ethics for use in family balancing. (See the next chapter for some of the ethics discussion of PGD for nonmedical purposes.) Regardless, this postconception method of gender selection is currently being done in select clinics inside and outside the United States, as described in this chapter, and PGD will probably grow as a sex selection method. It is an option that is available for your consideration.

CHAPTER

10

Gender Selection Today and in the Future

Gender selection has made amazing strides in the past decade—and this has basically occurred within the high-tech arena. Before these new technologies became available and publicly known, many people had never even guessed that choosing your baby's gender was an option. Many did not believe it was possible. Some are still not so sure.

Every day, more is being done in this area, and more women, or couples, are choosing to "chase" their gender dream. The demand is out there, and the possibilities are growing. If low-tech, at-home methods don't work for a couple, the next step can be medical technology: sperm spinning, MicroSort, artificial insemination, IVF, ICSI, PGD, you name it.

However, both MicroSort and PGD are still considered experimental. Some people are worried about health issues; some want to see more evidence, more examples of success stories, more medical acceptance by governmental bodies before advocating such new treatments. It is undoubtedly an area of concern for many—and those who have the most riding on the technology's health and safety are those of us who have done it. We want our children to be healthy and to grow up like any other child, no matter how conceived.

The MicroSort Track Record

What is the health record so far for MicroSort? Well, according to the clinical trial's website, neither the rate of spontaneous pregnancy loss nor the incidence of birth defects for MicroSort babies appears to differ from that of the general population. So far, the babies being born from the MicroSort process are as healthy as babies conceived elsewhere, according to the clinic's statistics, which it collects from every MicroSort pregnancy—both before birth and beyond.

"Based on the data so far, the likelihood of having a normal, healthy baby is not different from that of the general population," comments Dr. Daniel A. Potter of Huntington Reproductive Center in Laguna Hills, Calif., who is medical director for MicroSort West.

According to a report presented by Genetics & IVF Institute (GIVF) doctors at the 2003 annual meeting of the American College of Obstetricians and Gynecologists, the following was concluded: "Results confirmed MicroSort enrichment of X- and Y-bearing sperm populations that closely corresponded with baby gender. Fertilization, cleavage, miscarriage and pregnancy rates as well as incidence of major congenital malformations were comparable to those in literature reports utilizing unsorted sperm."

A sampling of MicroSort mothers I've talked to also shows a good health record so far for their children. And my daughter is healthy and developmentally normal (and looks perfect, I have to say!).

Professor Frank Comhaire, a physician who performs IVF with MicroSorted sperm in his clinic in Ghent, Belgium, has researched the use of fluorescence dye and laser-beam penetration of the sperm specimens in the MicroSort process. He comments, "So far, the proportion of major congenital abnormalities is 2.6 percent among the offspring after MicroSort cell sorting." This is reportedly in line with, or even better than, the statistics for the general birth population.

"In three out of five cases with such abnormalities, conception was achieved by IVF, and two cases had IUI," Dr. Comhaire continues. "Although the number of observations is far too small for final conclusions, the present data do not suggest an important increase in congenital abnormalities resulting from the procedure. Certainly more cases are needed. Since two out of the five cases with major congenital abnormalities had Down's syndrome, puncture of the amniotic fluid for cytogenetic evaluation is strongly recommended."

As for the future possibility of the MicroSort technology being licensed to fertility centers around the world, Dr. Comhaire comments, "I prefer the sorting to be performed in a center that has much experience, and that is seriously following up on treated couples in order to collect enough information to draw scientifically sound conclusions on efficacy and safety of the method."

The goals of the MicroSort program are to produce a certain amount of pregnancies, to show that efficacy and safety to the FDA and then to license the technology worldwide. Once MicroSort is out of FDA clinical trials, GIVF hopes to have laboratories with the sperm-sorting technology available all over the world. It is envisioned that patients will go to their local fertility center, where MicroSort will be licensed, and they'll provide a fresh semen sample to be sorted on the premises. This will be used for IUI or IVF, their choice.

"We hope that patients in every major city around the world will have access to this technology in the future," says Dr. Keith Blauer, GIVF MicroSort clinical director. Already two new MicroSort laboratories are planned to be open soon—a new facility in the Miami area scheduled for summer 2004, followed by a Chicago facility some time after that.

After MicroSort is out of FDA clinical trials, some things may change, such as the criteria for participation. Current criteria include the patients needing to be married, with the woman under 40, and their purpose for doing gender selection being either for family balancing or for avoiding a sex-linked disease in the family.

"The current inclusion and exclusion criteria are part of the FDA-approved clinical trial format. We would anticipate that women over the age of 39 would be able to participate after completion of the clinical trial," says Dr. Blauer.

And the costs of MicroSort? "We anticipate that improvements in technology will result in lower costs to the patient in the future," Dr. Blauer says.

Improvements in technology (especially in the IUI success rate) also may increase the number of couples who decide to attempt MicroSort.

"MicroSort is the only scientifically verifiable method of preconception gender selection. It is showing positive results after [hundreds of] pregnancies," states Dr. Potter. "For couples today who are considering options for having a family, especially those with chromosome-linked concerns, MicroSort gender selection is of serious interest. As the science continues to improve, we expect that MicroSort will become a routine part of family planning."

The Ethics of High-Tech Selection

Sex selection is not yet routine; it's far from that. The use of MicroSort and other types of gender selection technology is still controversial. There have been many discussions, and much written about, the ethics of such methods—of interfering with nature, of "playing God." What does the world in general think of gender selection technology? So far, the verdict is mixed.

"Sex selection is not legal in the United Kingdom at present if it involves using sorted sperm in IVF techniques to create an embryo—but not if it involves insemination with fresh sperm," a spokesperson from the Human Fertilisation and Embryology Authority, which licenses IVF clinics in the United Kingdom, told the BBC News in September 2003.

The Vatican, not surprisingly, is opposed to sex selection:

"Certain attempts to influence chromosomic or genetic inheritance are not therapeutic but are aimed at producing human beings selected according to sex or other predetermined qualities. These manipulations are contrary to the personal dignity of the human being and his or her integrity and identity. Therefore in no way can they be justified on the grounds of possible beneficial consequences for future humanity." This judgment was rendered in the *Instruction on Respect for Human Life in Its Origin and on the Dignity of Procreation* from the Vatican Congregation for the Doctrine of the Faith (1987).

So the Roman Catholic Church would be against MicroSort, not to mention the other gender selection technologies. As a result, couples who go through the procedure are more than likely to keep it a secret. Just about everybody I've talked to who has a MicroSort child, whether they're Catholic or not (and most are not), is secretive about sharing their offspring's origin with others. I only share my information with people who I feel will not judge me. It is a tough issue. Most MicroSorters believe it is their own business only, and no one else's. Or they are afraid of what people will think of them for using such an extreme method. We don't want to have to explain our reasons, our rationales, our emotions in wanting to influence the gender of our babies. We just know it is right for us. (For the "Islamic Point of View," see the adjacent box.)

Islamic Point of View

In Pakistan, the Salma & Kafeel Medical Centre's Infertility Services Ltd. has embraced gender selection. The fertility center obtained patent rights to Dr. Ronald Ericsson's sperm-spinning procedure for sex selection and touts the safety and efficacy of that method. They offer it for couples who are interested (see appendix for contact information).

"The issue of sex selection was put forward to the Pakistan Medical Association in July 2000," the center states. "According to our religious scholar, Dr. Khalid Mehmood Ghazi, choosing the gender of your child was within the parameters of Islamic injunctions. He further went on to say that any process that is performed with the husband and the wife is according to the Islamic injunctions."

Whether the average Islamic couple approves of gender selection remains to be seen, but this occurrence in Pakistan is an interesting development.

Some people say that gender selection is the start of ordering up "designer babies," that if we select the sex of our child today, then tomorrow it will be eye color, or some other characteristic. There is a lot of speculation about what other things people will try to influence in their future children. Television news shows that report on MicroSort like to group this technology with other opinions on "designer babies" in the same segment.

But from my experience and that of many other people, it appears that gender is far, far above any other characteristic when we think of what we want for our children. No one asks when a woman is pregnant, "Are you hoping for a blue-eyed child this time?" like they do about a boy or a girl. People who have always wanted a daughter, or a son, are not thinking along the same lines in dreams of a curly-haired child. To me, there is just no comparison.

Fortunately, the published professional opinion seems to be getting more supportive of gender selection technology.

According to an article in *The American Journal of Bioethics* (Winter 2001): "Safe and effective methods of preconception gender selection through flow cytometric separation of X- and Y-bearing sperm could greatly increase the use of gender selection by couples contemplating reproduction. Such a development raises ethical, legal and social issues about the impact of such practices on offspring, on sex ratio imbalances, and on sexism and the status of women." The writer, J.A. Robertson of the School of Law, University of Texas at Austin, "analyzes the competing interests in preconception gender selection, and concludes that its use to increase gender variety in a family, and possibly for selecting the gender of firstborn, might in many instances be ethically acceptable."

Back in 1994, the International Federation of Gynecology and Obstetrics stated, "Preconceptional sex selection can be justified on social grounds in certain cases for the objective of allowing children of the two sexes to enjoy the love and care of parents." (The organization also commented, "The use of preconceptional sex selection to avoid sex-linked genetic disorders is an indication that is completely justifiable on medical grounds.")

In May 2001, the Ethics Committee of the American Society for Reproductive Medicine (ASRM) made its report about preconception gender selection for nonmedical reasons in *Fertility and Sterility* (Vol. 75, No. 5). The committee concluded that if statistically valid clinical trials of the separation of X- and Y-producing sperm establish that the method is safe and effective, "the most prudent approach at present for the nonmedical use of these techniques would be to use them only for gender variety in a family, i.e., only to have a child of the gender opposite of an existing child or children."

That is what the majority of us who use MicroSort (those who do not need to produce a certain gender to avoid family genetic disorders) are doing it for: the family balancing aspect. We have a son or sons, and we want a daughter (or vice versa). We want to experience the gift of raising both boys and girls. We desire the opportunity to have the opposite-gender child to love and to raise.

The Ethics Committee continues, "If the social, psychological and demographic effects of those uses of preconception gender selection have been found acceptable, then other nonmedical uses of preconception selection might be considered."

So the future may have more plans for MicroSort.

If the well-respected ASRM is putting its OK on preconception gender selection technology, and the FDA approves MicroSort's clinical trials, we can expect to see couples all over the United States, and abroad, going into their local obstetrics office or fertility center and using sperm sorting services to plan their next baby.

"If flow cytometry or other methods of preconception gender selection are found to be safe and effective," states the Ethics Committee, "physicians should be free to offer preconception gender selection in clinical settings to couples who are seeking gender variety in their offspring if the couples [1] are fully informed of the risks of failure, [2] affirm that they will fully accept children of the opposite sex if the preconception gender selection fails, [3] are counseled about having unrealistic expectations about the behavior of children of the preferred gender, and [4] are offered the opportunity to participate in research to track and assess the safety, efficacy and demographics of preconception selection."

These are perfectly reasonable provisions, and ones that my husband and I were fully willing to accept when we began our

MicroSort journey. Soon more and more couples will join us in this new phase of medical science.

And once MicroSort is licensed all over the world, and more medical experts approve of it, will we mothers and fathers tell our friends, associates and relatives that we have used it? Perhaps.

Someday gender technology should become more commonplace, as more clinics perform the procedure and more people know about it. Already, PGD has grown as a gender selection technology, when before it was only performed by clinics for health purposes and most fertility centers refused to do it for family balancing. As more clinics become MicroSort providers, they may begin to consider PGD for gender selection as well, if they are skilled in the technology.

The Opinions on PGD

PGD, or gender selection *after* conception, may be a little harder for people to swallow. PGD as a sex selection technology is slowly starting to come around, and more clinics will now agree to do this for couples. However, embryo selection is definitely more controversial than sperm sorting—because, what becomes of the undesired embryos?

PGD for nonmedical purposes has been the subject of heated debate around the world. Individuals, organizations and governments of several countries have reviewed this issue and published statements on their opinions.

Although the American Society for Reproductive Medicine recently made a statement approving preconception gender technology such as MicroSort, its take on PGD for sex selection has not been as accepting. "Using preimplantation genetic diagnosis to determine the sex of an embryo conceived by IVF is ethically acceptable, but only if the aim is to avoid the transmission of genetic disorders. This is the only reason for choosing the sex of children that avoids the potential of 'gender bias,'" according to an ASRM panel report in the October 1999 issue of *Fertility and Sterility* (Vol. 72).

The panel's report focused on the use of PGD for gender selection and noted "the increasing attractiveness of pre-pregnancy sex selection." The panel issued the following in a press release: "This Ethics Committee Statement supports the use of [PGD] and sex selection to prevent the transmission of genetic diseases and discourages use of this technology for nonmedical family balancing or family planning purposes."

In a response to this ASRM statement, two individuals from the Murdoch Institute Ethics Program at Royal Children's Hospital in Melbourne, Australia, commented: "In its recent statement, the Ethics Committee of the American Society of Reproductive Medicine concluded that preimplantation genetic diagnosis for sex selection for non-medical reasons should be discouraged because it poses a risk of unwarranted gender bias, social harm, and results in the diversion of medical resources from genuine medical need. We critically examine the arguments presented against sex selection using preimplantation genetic diagnosis. We argue that sex selection should be available, at least within privately funded health care." J. Savulescu and E. Dahl wrote this in the September 2000 issue of *Human Reproduction* (Vol. 15).

And more recently in London, M. Pembrey of the Institute of Child Health at University College London, U.K., took a personal look at social sex selection by PGD, exploring this issue "from the dual perspectives of protecting the autonomy of the couple and the professional duty of care." As reported in *Reproductive Biomedicine Online* (2002, Vol. 4, No. 2), "It is concluded that sex selection by PGD is acceptable in certain circumstances."

Two medical experts, E.S. Sills and G.D. Palermo of Georgia Reproductive Specialists in Atlanta, Ga., reviewed this issue in the *Journal of Assisted Reproductive Genetics*

(September 2002, Vol. 19): "The promise of medical in-
novation has long evoked social commentary, particularly
when personal reproductive autonomy may be involved.
Development of the oral contraceptive, effective and safe
surgical sterilization, and later IVF and ICSI are among the
revolutionary developments where the initial reactions were
dubious but were accorded mainstream status with sufficient
clinical experience. In each instance, debate about the moral
and social implications of these treatments accompanied their
introduction into the medical marketplace.

"This pattern appears to be repeating itself in connection
with the use of preimplantation genetic diagnosis for elective
sex selection of human embryos. As with prior challenges
in reproductive medicine, the development of meaningful
'guidelines' for this latest controversy has proven to be a
contentious task. Indeed, the progression of ethics committee
reports from the American Society for Reproductive Medicine
seems to echo the ambivalence within society at large regarding this issue."

Undoubtedly, there is a lot of ambivalence out there. Ethical
issues surround PGD for sex selection, and it doesn't look like
there is going to be any general consensus in our society for a
while, if ever. Just as the public, and governmental officials,
debate what to do about the leftover, cryopreserved embryos
created from a regular IVF cycle, the idea of producing embryos
in order to select one gender over another is going to be part of
continued debate.

But one thing is for sure, and that is, no one in the field of
reproduction medicine is going to be able to ignore the possibilities of gender selection technology, including PGD. It is
available, it is effective and it will have to be addressed.

The European Society of Human Reproduction and
Embryology got into the issue recently, putting together an
ethics task force on the subject of PGD. The members set out
a recommended multidisciplinary approach to the application

of PGD, including consideration of "fundamental ethical principles, specific problems in cases of high genetic risk, and PGD for aneuploidy screening, HLA typing and sex selection for non-medical reasons" (*Human Reproduction*, March 2003, Vol. 18). We will have to see where this recommended approach goes.

Whether or not it is offered for sex selection, PGD is going to continue to be a reproductive technology on the cutting edge, as more research is done in this area and more clinics get involved.

Fertility Centers of Illinois (FCI), with several locations in the Chicago area, is one of the MicroSort collaborators (see contact information for Dr. Angeline Beltsos in appendix). These clinics also offer the latest in PGD technology and are a proponent of research in this area, especially for women at risk of having a genetically abnormal fetus. "The early worldwide experience with PGD is full of promise," FCI comments. "Work is still needed to clarify the appropriate role of preimplantation genetic diagnosis in many situations. Many ethical considerations will certainly be encountered as the potential uses for this technology are broadened. It promises to expand the treatment choices available for couples."

The Future

We will have to wait to see what is next for gender selection technology. PGD probably has more hurdles to pass in gaining public acceptance for family balancing than the MicroSort and Ericsson methods do. But all of the sex selection technologies still have a long way to go before becoming a routine part of family planning (not to mention the fact that the costs need to come down).

More people every year are becoming familiar with the concept of sex selection, however. And the question often arises: If high-tech gender selection becomes common throughout the world, would there be a prevalence of selecting for one particular gender over another? Would the planet's birth sex ratio be seriously altered? This is always an issue brought up in discussions about sex preselection, especially by its opponents.

Evidence from MicroSort and Ericsson patient samples shows that in the United States, baby girls are the leading request from couples undergoing sperm separation. In addition, those who do PGD often are seeking daughters, especially if they're worried about passing on a sex-linked genetic disorder. And if women are going to subject themselves and their bodies to the rigors of IVF, it's usually because *they* have the preference for a particular offspring gender—and that's usually girls.

However, in other parts of the world, especially in underdeveloped areas, it would be the reverse.

"In most less developed societies, parents seem to have preference for sons rather than daughters," according to Lakshmi K. Raut in the *Journal of Qualitative Economics* (January 1996, Vol. 12). "The preference for sons may be rooted purely in taste and cultural values or it could be the outcome of some economic calculations. For instance, sons generally stay with their parents while daughters are married off to another household, so that sons tend to provide better support in old age as well as augment current household income."

In the mid-1990s, Peter Liu and G. Alan Rose of the London Gender Clinic studied the social characteristics of more than 800 couples attending their clinic for sex preselection. The patients had an ethnic origin of 57.8 percent Indian, 32.0 percent European, 3.6 percent Chinese and 6.8 percent other. The average age of the women was 34 years.

The results of the study indicated that "Asian and Middle Eastern couples overwhelming wanted boys, whereas European couples showed a slight preference for girls," according to Liu and Rose in the journal *Human Reproduction*

(1995, Vol. 10, No. 4). "These results suggest that, given certain guidelines, sex selection is unlikely to lead to a serious distortion of the sex ratio in Britain and other Western societies, but may need careful monitoring in other parts of the world."

The researchers give their opinion of the reasons: "In countries like India, China and Korea, boys are highly prized, mainly for economic reasons, although the ability to carry on the family name is also important. The financial hardship of raising girls in these countries has led to the abandonment of female children and the widespread use of abortion and even infanticide in favor of boys.

"In other societies like the Middle East, the preference for boys is probably more for religious-cultural than economic reasons," write the researchers.

And in Europe and the United States? "In Western societies, the motivation for sex selection is less understood and is probably more of a personal nature than anything else."

I can attest to that, as my gender quest was definitely one of a very personal nature. As other women I have met (harking from the U.S., Canada, Europe and Australia) will agree, there was just an unexplainable longing, a desire to fill a "void" in the family, an unending hope to have a little girl. This is the demand that high-tech gender selection meets. At least in the Western world.

In America, "women are primarily the ones who decide whether or not to have another child. Those of age to reproduce have a much different opinion of themselves and their position in society as did their mothers and grandmothers," Dr. Ronald Ericsson explains. "Therefore, they are motivated to have daughters as they see a bright future for them. More females than males graduate from high school, enroll and graduate from college. These young woman have the ability to be economically independent and not marry. Those who choose to have a child and not marry also prefer daughters.

Many women state that they want the mother-daughter relationship that they had with their mothers. The era of wanting a first-born male is gone not to return."

Well, whether that is true in the United States and other Western countries, we have yet to find out, as high-tech gender selection begins to spread its wings.

When Dr. Comhaire of Belgium was asked about the future consequences of gender sperm sorting, if it were to be available all over the world, he commented, "I am aware of the preferences of the European couples, where the majority request sperm selection to enhance the probability of delivering a daughter (possibly because of the constant 'excess' of boys born; the male over female ratio being 1.05). In China and India, the pressure on women may, in fact, decrease as soon as the mother has delivered a boy. However, the principle of offering the technique exclusively to those couples who already have at least one child, and desire a child of the opposite gender, should prevent sexism and severe imbalance in the population."

When asked about possible legal restrictions on the use of nonmedical gender selection, Dr. Comhaire states, "What is nonmedical? If medicine would be restricted to exclusively treating (and preventing) genetic diseases, then most of our medical work would stop! Medicine also aims at promoting 'health,' both physical and mental. Family balancing may improve the mental well-being of particular couples. I am convinced that sexuality and reproduction are purely private matters and these should not be interfered with, provided three conditions are fulfilled."

Those conditions are—

• The absence of negative effects on society.
• The absence of any negative effects on the existing family.
• The absence of hazardous side effects on the offspring.

"If these conditions are satisfied, there is no need for paternalistic legal restrictions or interference," Dr. Comhaire comments.

If more medical doctors think this way, then high-tech gender selection has a strong future. Who knows what will happen in the upcoming years, as sex selection expands and becomes more common in our communities. Will the natural sex ratio be skewed in the world? I hope not. But I also hope that we don't lose this wonderful opportunity to fulfill our dreams. Stay tuned.

Conclusion

The demand for gender selection is out there, and it's not going to go away. There seems to have been a major increase in this demand in recent years, and governments and reproductive health organizations are starting to discuss it. The topic is getting noticed, it is getting addressed, and there will continue to be many debates about sex selection (both before conception and after). And more couples are going to attempt it.

When I started on my quest for a daughter in the 1990s, I thought I was alone. As I explained in this book's preface, no one around me could understand the need for a particular gender in one's children. Those I mentioned it to, including my own extended family, could not relate. As always, I typically was told that all that mattered was the health of the baby. I agreed to a point—I definitely wanted healthy children. But if I could do something to bring about a daughter, I hoped for that, too. What is wrong with that?

I quietly did my own research, I met up with other women on Internet bulletin boards and I found a whole, underground world of people like me hoping to do "gender determination"—some people who had already tried, some who were in the midst of a current cycle trying for a daughter or son, and some who were just in the planning stages for their future baby. I met women who had just given birth to their second or third son, and though they were overjoyed at the new life they had created, they were still hoping for the next child, a daughter. Others were, at the time, just finding out the sex of their current pregnancy at ultrasound, and they found themselves typing through tears on their computer, pouring out their feelings to others who would understand their disappointment.

I found I was not alone. Other women felt the way I did, were fixated on trying to conceive a daughter for their family, and in our "virtual" online world, we didn't have to feel embarrassed, ashamed or guilty. We had allies in our search for answers. And these allies were all over the world. I met women from across the country, and from Canada, Europe and Australia, who all felt like I did. And I really was encouraged by this. I made online friends with these other women, sometimes meeting them in person, and we told each other things we might not tell our friends "IRL" (in real life). When we had any conception, pregnancy or childbirth news, these online friends were often one of the first to find it out. For some, we were each other's lifelines.

I know that this need will continue to be there for other women (and men) after me—there will always be people who are hoping to do something to influence the gender of their next child, or maybe even their first child. And I am hoping that this book will help them, as I hope it has helped you. A generation after my daughter was born, I know others will be looking for some answers. Years after I checked out my first fertility book from the library or searched for "sex selection" on the World Wide Web, there will be couples wondering about these same topics. Decades after the online bulletin boards were first created and used by so many around the world, people everywhere will be making decisions and going to the Web for support.

I find that this is an often hidden desire, to preselect our child's gender. But in every generation, there are going to be people who have this same passion. Rather than suppress this passion, or fixation, maybe they can do something about it.

I hope that this book will be a resource for those of you who also feel this desire, and I want to let you know that if you feel the same way, you are not alone. For years I had this image of a little girl in a family photo, and now she is here in flesh and blood, all wispy blond hair and big smiles. Those family portraits have now been shot, the holiday dresses have been bought, I no longer feel sad in children's clothing stores. I used to look longingly at the girls section—now I can shop there. The first time I went to purchase a little dress and hairbows for my daughter, I almost welled up with tears. The moment had been such a long time coming...

Maybe your dream of pink or blue can come true, too.

In the preceding chapters I have tried to cover every sex selection method I've heard about, and researched, and to give you honest answers about each one and what is being said about it. And on the next pages, I include an appendix for you to use for more information: check out a support board, read another book, look into a clinic. I hope it helps! I wish you luck in chasing your dream.

Appendix

Here are resources and contact details to provide you with more information about gender selection in your journey for a girl or a boy.

Clinics, Medical Centers and Physicians

Angeline N. Beltsos, M.D. (MicroSort collaborator)
Fertility Centers of Illinois
2825 N. Halsted
Chicago, IL 60659
(773) 472-4400
www.fcionline.com

Cooper Center for IVF (collaborating MicroSort clinic)
8002 Greentree Commons
Marlton, NJ 08053
(856) 751-5250 or 751-5575
www.ccivf.com

Frank Comhaire, M.D. (MicroSort collaborator)
Fertility Clinic Congreslaan, 6
Gent, Belgium B-900
+32 475 618555

Michael T. Drouin, M.D.
(Ericsson Method sex selection center)
Women's Health Center
287 Main Street, Suite 201
Lewiston, ME 04240
(207) 795-7180
michaeld@megalink.net

Energy Health Centre
(Clinic with gender preselection services)
43 Marne Street
South Yarra
VIC 3141
Australia
+613 9866 8667
www.energyhealthcentre.com

The Fertility Institutes
(Clinic with MicroSort, PGD services)
18370 Burbank Blvd., Suite 414
Tarzana, CA
(818) 776-8700
TZFertility@aol.com
www.fertility-docs.com/fertility_gender.phtml

Gametrics Limited
(developers of the Ericsson Albumin Method)
HC 69, Box 50
Alzada, MT 59311
(307) 878-4494 or (915) 364-2645
ericsson@childselect.com
gametrics@childselect.com
www.childselect.com

Genetics & IVF Institute (developers of MicroSort)
3020 Javier Road
Fairfax, VA 22031
(703) 698-7355 or (800) 552-4363
givf@givf.com
www.givf.com

Huntington Reproductive Center (MicroSort West)
23961 Calle de la Magdalena
Suite 541
Laguna Hills, CA 92653
(949) 472-9446 or (866) 472-4483 (toll-free)
www.havingbabies.com

Dr. Peter Liu (MicroSort collaborator)
London Gender Clinic
359 Hendon Way
London NW4 3LY
United Kingdom
+44(0)20-8202-2900
pksliu@aol.com
www.sexselection.co.uk

Malpani Infertility Clinic (IVF/PGD center)
Jamuna Sagar
Shahid Bhagat Singh Road
Colaba
Bombay 400 005
India
91-22-2151065, 2151066 or 2150223
malpani@bigfoot.com
www.drmalpani.com

MicroSort® — Division of the Genetics & IVF Institute
3015 Williams Drive, Suite 101
Fairfax, VA 22031
(703) 876-3897 or (800) 277-6607
Collaborator Services: (703) 876-3899
microsort@givf.com
www.microsort.com

Salma & Kafeel Medical Centre Infertility Services
(Ericsson Method sex selection center)
H. #11, St. #54, F-7/4
Islamabad-Pakistan
051-2276143-2873412
skmc@comsats.net.pk

Andrew Y. Silverman, M.D.
(Ericsson Method sex selection center)
12 Greenridge Ave., Suite 400
White Plains, NY 10605
(914) 761-4622
info@gender-preselect.com

Ronald G. Zack, M.D.
(Ericsson Method sex selection center)
Midwest Fertility & Sex Selection Center
55 North Pond Drive, Suite #2
Walled Lake, MI 48390
(248) 624-3366
mwfertility@htdconnect.com
www.selectagender.com/

******

Information Websites

Baby Center (Determining Sex message board)
http://bbs.babycenter.com/board/preconception/
gettingpregnant/

ChinaGold (Chinese lunar method and survey results)
www.chinagold.com/baby.htm

GeoCities Gender Determination (information website)
www.geocities.com/genderdetermination

In-Gender (information website and survey results)
www.in-gender.com/ig/

iVillage's Parent Soup
(Gender Determination message board)
http://messageboards.ivillage.com/iv-psgender

Preconception.com
(Choosing the Sex of Your Baby message board)
http://interact.iparenting.com//postlistphp?Cat=&Board=
choosesex

******

Books and Publications on Gender Selection and Fertility

Boy or Girl?
The Definitive Work on Sex Selection
By Dr. Elizabeth Whelan
Published by Pocket Books, rev. ed. March 1991

How to Choose the Sex of Your Baby:
The Method Best Supported by Scientific Evidence
By Landrum B. Shettles, M.D., and David M. Rorvik
Published by Doubleday, rev. ed. January 1997

The Preconception Gender Diet
By Sally Langendoen and William Proctor
Published by M. Evans & Co., April 1982

"Preconception Selection of Sex in Man"
Israel Journal of Medical Science, Vol. 17 (1981)
By J. Stolkowski and J. Choukroun

Taking Charge of Your Fertility:
The Definitive Guide to Natural Birth Control, Pregnancy
Achievement, and Reproductive Health
By Toni Weschler
Published by Quill, rev. ed. November 2001

Note: All of the information above is just a sampling of the available resources, not a complete or exhaustive list.

Index

Printed in the United States
21495LVS00001BA/235

9 781593 301484